Hungry

TRUST YOUR BODY
AND FREE YOUR MIND
AROUND FOOD

♥

TARA WHITNEY

Published by Birch Tree Press

Cover and book design and artwork: Domini Dragoone
Editors: Jennifer Hartmann and Christina Roth
Photo of author: Raya On Assignment
Cover photo: © Seb Ra/iStock

Library of Congress Cataloging-in-Publication Data is available.

ISBN: 978-1-7339096-0-0 (paperback)
ISBN: 978-1-7339096-1-7 (e-book)

Printed in the United States of America

DEDICATION

*For every woman who has had enough of hating her body
and feeling so out of control around food, and is ready
to boldly and courageously love and accept herself.*

Contents

PART FOUR – JOURNEY

HUNGRY

Introduction

Dearest reader,

In your hands you have the start of a new conversation around food, your body image, and a sense of your own self-worth. This may be hard for you to believe, as there are thousands of books you could be reading, or have already read, about these topics. You could be reading about gluten-free, sugar-free, or dairy-free diets or the latest trending diet. You could be reading about those with eating disorders and how they overcame them. With the positive body image movement that has risen over the past decade, you could be learning how to stop hating your body. There are thousands of these conversations for you to engage in.

Over the past three-plus decades, I have been part of these conversations. Without a doubt, they have helped me create the content in the pages to follow. At a very young age, I made it my mission to find a way to fix my struggles with food and permanently be thin. I educated myself on a huge variety of diets. I followed low-fat diets and ate frozen Weight Watchers dinners. I ate only fruit in the morning. I juiced and stopped eating meat, dairy, and fish.

And then I went in the other direction. I cut out grains and gluten, filled my plate with steak, and ate an avocado a day. I had thoroughly researched each of these diets before I jumped into them. They all had strong and well-documented research to back up their claims of improved health and weight loss. Their before-and-after success stories each revealed better-dressed, more confident, and happier people as a result of their weight loss. The promise was so alluring that I always saw myself in these pictures, imagining myself in skinny jeans, feeling the sense of satisfaction and confidence I so craved. As I went from diet to diet, I always put my faith and trust in those experts—both the dieters and researchers. I chose to follow them because of the documented success they offered. I wanted to be my own success story. But I rarely was. At least not for long.

OVEREATERS ANONYMOUS: RESTRICT AND CONTROL

I was first exposed to dieting when I was eight. My brother and I joined our mother at her Overeaters Anonymous (OA) meetings because we were too young to stay at home by ourselves. OA uses a similar approach to Alcoholics Anonymous, following a twelve-step program that claims to help members abstain from sugar and white flour.

My brother and I would sit in the back of the room, outside the circle the members sat in. Men and women of all shapes and sizes shared their own stories about food and abstinence. New members would often cry, which always caught our attention. Veteran members shared their success and spoke of working the "steps." During each meeting, my brother and I heard declarations repeated out loud in unison. They stated their powerlessness over food and asked God to guide them in overcoming their powerlessness.

My mother kept a spiral-bound notebook on the corner of the kitchen table in which she diligently recorded what she ate. Her white food scale sat on the left side of the kitchen sink and got frequent use. I overheard her on the phone every evening, sharing with someone her food plan for the next day. This person was her sponsor.

I was so educated in OA, I convinced my childhood best friend to diet with me, OA-style. She and I would be each other's sponsors, and we would follow a food plan. Just a few days after our new diet began, I visited my grandmother. She had just bought my favorite cookie of all time: Fig Newtons. I couldn't resist. One led to another, and before I knew it, I had eaten six. Thankfully, I knew how to fix this. I called my dear friend and confessed. But she didn't know OA, and she didn't quite know which step I needed to work. Instead, I heard a hint of frustration in her voice. I was asking her for an answer that she didn't have. I hung up the phone and went back to the kitchen to eat another cookie. I knew how to diet, and I knew how to fail at dieting.

Some of the first conversations I was part of around food and weight loss were in church basements and hospital conference rooms. I heard that I had to restrict, control, and limit what I ate and how I ate it. Certain foods—in particular, pastas, sugary treats, and ice cream—were to be avoided at all costs. I knew that sacrifice and persistence were needed to achieve abstinence, including diligently planning meals, measuring and weighing chicken breast and salad, and reporting what I ate to someone else.

My mother didn't intend for me to be part of this conversation. My brother and I were innocent bystanders, breathing in each word like secondhand smoke. It would take me decades to become aware of the assumptions and beliefs I had made my own, to loosen their grip on me and ultimately release myself from them.

NEVER ENOUGH

One late Sunday morning when I was eleven, I lay on my living room couch watching old Elvis movies. I was by myself. My mother was working, and my stepfather and brother had taken off for the day. I walked into the kitchen to make myself a sandwich, added chips and cookies to my plate, and returned to the couch. After I finished what was on my plate, I wanted more. More chips. More cookies. More chips. More cookies. More. More. I made so many trips to the kitchen.

When there were no More left, I was stunned. What just happened? I didn't know. My belly was so full I could barely move, and my mind was so empty I couldn't come up with any answers. I only knew how shameful I felt. No one could find out what I did. I wouldn't mention a word to anyone.

If that had been my first and last binge, I would not be having this conversation with you. You know it wasn't. When I was in my early teens, I'd come home from school to an empty house. I ate rhythmically: one cookie, then another. And another. There was no stopping until the cookies were gone. I'd no longer feel stunned, but I would feel the same disgust and shame as when I ate until I felt sick. What did I do then? I would make myself go for a run. Every step I would take would be a constant reminder of my mistake. My overfilled belly was too painful for me to ignore. This was my punishment and the price I needed to pay.

DESPERATE AND EXHAUSTED

Over time, my conversation around food and weight loss turned into one question. One that I constantly asked myself. How could I stop eating so much so I could finally lose weight?

I was determined to find the answer. I joined programs, saw therapists, and paid good money to work with coaches. I was trying to do it right, based on everything I knew to do, yet I was still overeating and binging. Exercise was the other part of the equation. Controlling how much I ate was hard. Controlling how far I ran and how long I worked out at the gym was easier.

And quite honestly, I just ran in circles. There was always more weight to come off, yet it never did. Considering how hard I was trying, I was convinced something was wrong with me. How else could I answer this persistent question? I was doing everything that I thought would help me lose weight. But it didn't work.

Over time, I grew weary. I had a vision of me on a gerbil wheel, working tirelessly but not making any progress. No matter how hard I ran, I stayed in the same place. When I would go to bed with an achy belly from a binge, I was desperate to try anything. The next morning, believing the day ahead of me would be different would give me hope. Hope that I could eat perfectly. Hope that I could drop a jean size and finally feel good about myself.

While I was on the gerbil wheel, I suspected something wasn't quite right. I knew I wanted to stop abusing my body. I knew I wanted to stop feeling sick from eating so much. My drive to find a new understanding of my struggles with food and my body was insatiable. I recognized the discomfort of despising, overfilling, and starving my body, and I hated it.

Stepping off the gerbil wheel didn't happen after reading just one book or participating in one program that promised me a different solution. But you probably suspected that. Our bookshelves are filled with books that promise us magic but only deliver us to the same place we started. I can only tell you of the process I was taking as I found a new way. I became aware of my thinking and what I was believing. As I opened my eyes and ears, I became really skeptical and curious of all the outside forces that impacted how I felt about my body, how I ate, and my own well-being. Ultimately, there was one side of a conversation that was happening, and I had to be very mindful which ones were the right ones for me to engage in. Stepping off the gerbil wheel meant that I started having new conversations. Like the one I'm about to have with you.

There came a point when I concretely noticed the freedom I had created for myself around food. I knew how to choose to eat foods that fueled and nourished me. And I was trusting my own body to know how much was enough, to know when my body was simply satisfied. Was I doing it 100 percent of the time with exact precision? Of course not. Spoiler alert: perfectionism is not our way off the gerbil wheel.

Truthfully, when I found space in my mind from food and confidence in myself around how to eat, I wanted to leave my whole history of disordered eating, emotional eating, and overeating behind. I considered burning every self-help and diet book I had ever purchased. Or at least donate them to a thrift shop for some other struggling woman to purchase on discount. As I contemplated doing this, I realized that I knew the woman who would want to buy the books I had read. I had a vision of her knocking quietly on my front door. It was a knock I couldn't ignore, because I knew she wasn't going away. My temptation to ignore her was my way of dismissing my own struggles and the process I had uncovered. A small part of me wanted to stay hidden. If I had, I would have been undermining myself and giving into any residual shame around my past experiences with food.

I knew she didn't need a single one of my books. She didn't need another diet or another therapist. She didn't need a gym membership to motivate her or a Weight Watchers leader to tell her to stay on track. She needed to hear the truth. I realized this over five years ago. Since then, I've opened the door to sharing my own journey, tools, and methods with women like her as their transformational coach. I knew it would be selfish if I didn't. All my trials and inner conflicts would have been wasted if I couldn't guide other women to move beyond their struggles, to be the support I wish I'd had.

I'll be sharing with you some collective stories of my clients on these pages. In some cases, their stories are a blend of a few individual experiences. In all cases, the names I share are fictitious.

This new conversation I discovered years ago will introduce you to a dear and loving friend: your body! This new conversation will allow you to experience food in a whole new way. This new conversation will start to change your mindset around your feelings. These conversations are opportunities, opportunities to connect with your own wisdom and divine intelligence. They will bring you back to yourself. Now, that's a conversation worth having.

Ready? Let's chat.

Empty

♥

PART ONE

CHAPTER ONE

Something Is Missing

When we struggle with food, we are truly hungry. A deep hunger that's hard to recognize. No amount of food, decadent dark chocolate cake, fresh, hot New York pizza, or any gluten-free, sugar-free, dairy-free dish will satisfy this hunger. We know—we've tried to fulfill our hunger with food, and it's still not quelled.

Our hunger has been so present in our lives, and we've known something isn't quite right. We've known the feeling of never doing our diets well enough. We've known the feeling of losing weight and feeling self-conscious, like we are in someone else's skin, trying to be someone we are not. We know the gerbil wheel of trying to lose weight, like we've been sentenced to keep spinning because we believe it's our only choice.

The void and emptiness touches us personally, so we inevitably can also witness it in our culture. Eating disorder incidences have skyrocketed in the past two decades.[1] Depression, especially among young people between the ages of twelve and seventeen, are on a significant rise.[2] The already massive weight loss industry continues to grow at a steady rate, with no signs of slowing down.

SKINNY AND INSECURE

Four months after joining Weight Watchers (this was after the birth of my first child) I lost over fifteen pounds. Friends, coworkers, and family praised my thinness. I always felt their eyes on my body, taking a few extra moments examining me. It was as if they had to make sure my body, the thinner one, was really me.

After so much hard work and focus, you'd think I would celebrate my success and my leaner body. Instead, I was afraid that I'd lose what I had. As if I'd received a gift I didn't deserve, I was waiting for it to be taken away. I was worried I'd gain the weight back. I was afraid of letting down those around me, the ones who praised me and were so impressed with my achievements. I felt like a fraud waiting to expose herself. My thinner body was a cover-up, and soon everyone would see the real me. The one who wasn't able to permanently keep the weight off. The one who weighed more.

This fear is common for people who have lost weight. My clients have shared that they have had at least one time in their lives when they dropped the weight and were fitting into smaller clothes they had never worn before. Yet instead of feeling secure and confident in their skinnier body, they kept looking over their shoulder, like they were the lead runner in a race. They kept anticipating if and when they would be caught by the runner behind them. Losing weight didn't leave them satisfied; it left them worried they would gain the weight back. And they each did.

NEVER ENOUGH

When I was dieting and restricting how I ate, a big part of me believed I could always do it better. At the end of each day, I would run through a mental checklist of how I did against my current diet. It could have been paleo, vegan, vegetarian, or keto. It didn't matter. How I ate that day wasn't good enough. For me, dieting was trying to reach a standard I couldn't quite attain, no matter how hard I tried. It had to be perfect, but never was.

As a young girl, watching my mother diet and try to lose weight gave me one possible path to follow. However, I didn't just see her in her own version of her skinny jeans; I also witnessed all her hard work. She weighed, measured, and recorded every snack and meal she ate. Food was something to try to manage perfectly and control.

My relationship with food meant work and worry. And at the end of the day, no matter how well I did, I was never happy with myself. I was never satisfied. When I watched other women so relaxed around food, I would be in awe. They left food on their plate, casually mentioned to me they forgot to eat a meal, and ordered food I had forbidden myself at a restaurant. I was envious and longed for something I didn't think was possible for me.

DIETING ALONE

I wished I could have been invisible when I would bring my own special dishes to restaurants or parties. On my weight loss quest, I needed to have with me the food that I was allowed to eat. I'd secretly pray that no one would notice, but they always did. While on a juice cleanse, I'd quietly tell the waitress that I would only have water and then drink my green smoothie while everyone I was with ate their pasta, chicken, and breadsticks. I would try to casually brush off their comments, but not eating like everyone else set me apart from my family, friends, and coworkers. I was different. I couldn't afford to eat like everyone else. I was on the outside, and there was a distance between me and them.

NEGLECTED FEELINGS

It took me years to realize my own patterns around food when I ate because of stress, sadness, and loneliness. After overeating or binging, my mind immediately searched for a solution for me to stop this destructive behavior. I was only worried about weight gain, and my guilt and shame drove me to find a way to burn the calories I had just consumed. I wasn't concerned with how badly I felt. My weight and concern of gaining any amount of it kept me distracted. Eating half a bag of Hershey's Kisses didn't take away my sadness. I just got to focus on something else. Meanwhile, my sadness was still there, unattended.

We've been hungry for something more than any amount of food or weight loss can offer. We've been hungry for a different way to live. In fact, our relationship with food, our bodies, and how we feel has only increased our true hunger. Let's talk about where this emptiness began, as it came long before we were even born.

CHAPTER TWO

Messages: Hungry to Be Enough

Thin women are happy, attractive, and successful.

Chances are high that you agree with this statement. Or you're at least aware the belief is held by many, even if you don't hold it for yourself. Before we say more, we need to understand where this statement came from, who keeps saying it, and the real impact it's had on us and our ability to nourish and love our bodies.

A PIVOTAL CHOICE

I grew up loving softball. And I was quite good. John Fogerty's "Centerfield" must have been written for me, and I listened to it often. Softball came to me easily and effortlessly, whether I was in the outfield or the batter's box. A few months into my freshman year in college, I was invited to try out for the softball team. That was a big deal at my state university.

At the first practice, I scanned each player's body. I saw their broad shoulders and thick thighs. They were strong athletes, no question. But they weren't thin enough, cute enough, small enough. They weren't feminine. No blond hair. No ponytails and lip gloss. I felt a cruel disgust.

I didn't want to be part of this team. What I really wanted was to run far away and leave them and my softball-playing days behind.

I told the softball coach that the time commitment was too much for me. I told her I had to focus on my classes and schoolwork. She understood, as far as I could tell. She didn't detect my cover-up for the lie it was.

A few months later, I walked into another coach's office and asked her for a summer training schedule. I ran cross-country for two seasons, and we raced against some big competitive schools. I ran, literally and figuratively, toward and with the women I wanted to be like. These women were strong athletes, no question. But more importantly, they were pretty and feminine. And, of course, thin.

At nineteen, I held the belief that thin women were happy, attractive, and successful, and it led me to dismiss my innate talents and skills. I played down my passions because what I loved was dangerous. Being with athletic women who weren't thin was a cruel fate in my mind. And most of those softball players weren't skinny or skinny enough. If I were on their team, it meant I was like them. Not feminine. Not small. Not pretty. Not skinny. I couldn't do it.

This was the late 1980s, and this statement about women was already firmly planted inside me. Where did I hear it, and who told it to me?

AN UNDETECTED GAS

Our minds are like sponges, soaking up images and conversations all around us. We don't consciously take it all in; instead, information gets stored in our unconscious brains. Beliefs are what we know to be true, not necessarily fact, but instead an interpretation of experiences, assumptions, observations, and conclusions.

The statement, "Thin women are happy, attractive and successful," is a long-held belief that we've formed in our minds and has been largely undetected for decades and decades. It's like a gas in your home that can't be smelled or seen. We've been blanketed in this message, this belief. Once a belief is formed, we look for information—or evidence, if you will—that confirms our belief. We see and hear evidence that this belief is true in magazines, on TV, and in conversations with our coworkers.

We can't question something we can't see. It's so prevalent, we can't even point to it. Believing all or parts of this message about women is all we know, it's all our mothers knew, and it's all our grandmothers knew.

This message has weaved its way into the fabric of our culture, particularly in the realm of entertainment.

TV entertains us. TV offers us the assumptions made by Hollywood, playing out in the shows they create, actors they cast, and lines they write. We see very thin actresses living glamorous lives. They are wealthy, sexy, and desirable.Where the message packs the punch is often in the desirable personality traits of the actresses.

The Solid Gold dancers mesmerized me before I was even a teenager. I would sit intently in my grandmother's La-Z-Boy chair, taking in their long legs and fishnet stockings. Even if I didn't have words for it at the time, I knew they were talented and sexy.

Daisy from The Dukes of Hazzard also captured my attention. She could fearlessly drive a car, get herself out of trouble, and charm her way out of any situation—all while wearing her infamous cutoff denim shorts and tied flannel shirt. My young and impressionable mind saw Daisy as happy, fun, and pretty. She could drive a Jeep like a badass (although I didn't know that word at the time), and I loved her sass and rebellious spirit.

I didn't just see Daisy's and the Solid Gold dancers' thin bodies and beauty; I also saw something I desired for myself.

Hollywood masterfully connected the two things for me in my mind.

These are just two examples, but there are millions of impressions, assumptions, values, and ideals around beauty and attractiveness we encounter every time we turn on the TV.

A PARADE OF BEAUTY

It would be inaccurate to say that beauty contests were the start of when women's bodies were judged and objectified. It's been happening for centuries, in all parts of the world.

However, in the United States, the Miss America pageant is one marked phenomenon that first evaluated young women's physical attributes in 1921. Margaret Gorman was the first crowned Miss America, competing on a popular boardwalk in Atlantic City, New Jersey. At the age of sixteen and weighing 108 pounds, she was awarded the Golden Mermaid trophy and crowned the most beautiful bathing girl in America.

For nearly a century, Miss America has been evaluating contestants for qualities that they deem worthy of the queen of beauty. For example, grace and a commanding presence are measured through contestants' swimsuits and evening gowns.[3]

Miss America pageants, Miss Universe competitions, Victoria's Secret Angels shows, and fashion designers' shows parade women across their stages and runways. Along with the judges, we evaluate these women, rank them, and assess their beauty. The bodies we see are homogenous, each thin. We don't see a wide range of body sizes and shapes on these stages. We don't think to ask why, because we know. No one had to use words to tell us. This is another form of the undetected gas that we've been taking in. The message is clear. It's much more than, "Thin women are beautiful." It's, "Beauty only comes in one size." It's thin. And because we rarely see a variety of body sizes and shapes, we conclude that if a woman has a bigger body, she must not be beautiful.

SELLING HAPPY, RICH, AND SEXY

No matter the product, thin and attractive models represent what companies are selling. Thin women are enjoying wine with close girlfriends, catching the eyes of men while wearing certain shoes, and receiving the loving affection of their significant others while wearing diamond necklaces. All that we desire comes along with thinness: friendship, attention, love, and affection. We aren't just seeing thin women; we are watching them live a life everyone wants to live.

Marketers are masterful at selling to us our desires. We are being sold on the experience of owning the watch, not the watch itself. A watch commercial won't share its fine technology, where it was built, or how it was made. Instead, we see a beautiful, elegantly dressed model wearing the watch. Thanks to persuasive marketing, owning an expensive watch can make us feel sexy and beautiful. At least that's the way we see it.

If we aren't being sold on our desires, we are being sold on how our problems can be solved.

Marketers know how to get us to buy their products, and it includes hiring actresses and models painting for us a picture of how our life will be better and our problems will be solved if we purchase those products. These models are always thin.

Take the product itself out of the equation, and we consciously or unconsciously draw a connection in our minds: happiness, wealth, and sexiness is always accompanied by thin women.

Societal messages have evolved dramatically in the last century. In the past, they were communicated on printed newspapers and from words spoken in churches, classrooms, and coffee shops. Now, messages fly at us with great persistence and frequency when we pick up our phones, read our emails, watch our favorite sports teams, go to movie theaters, and flip through magazines in grocery store checkout lines.

In the 1970s it was estimated that we received about fifty brand images a day. Now, that estimate has increased one hundred times. We now carry around the messaging center in our purse and receive over five thousand messages a day.[4]

The result? We've become desensitized. These messages are no longer unusual or dramatic. We just see these messages as the truth, and there are too many of them to even question or dismiss.

OUT-OF-REACH AND FICTITIOUS IDEALS

Over the past twenty years, the average women's size has increased from size 8 to size 12. During this same time period, the average model size has decreased from size 8 to size 0.[5]

When we pick up a fashion magazine, go to the movie theater, or watch a show on Netflix, we are witnessing women's bodies that are vastly smaller than our own.

We are well aware that photographs and digital technology modify and alter any picture, and the glamour industry has been altering pictures for decades. The modifications may be slight or significant. No matter. The pictures we see of models and actresses are altered to smooth skin, brighten teeth, and remove scars or tattoos. Physically, bodies are altered according to the wishes of whoever is doing the altering. Larger breasts or smaller breasts. Six-pack abs. Thinner thighs.

We are constantly seeing pictures of women who don't really exist. We are shown a view of perfection that's so far from our own reality.

SPREADING THE MESSAGE

Chances are, you've received comments from people about your weight. Or you've made your own comments on others' weight. No one is immune to this undetected gas. We've all been exposed to it to one degree or another. These comments often hold the code that carries the underlying belief "thin women are happy, attractive, and successful." That's what happens with embedded societal conditioning. The message has unique and distinct ways of permeating into our lives. For example:

- Your college roommate went on a diet and lost twenty pounds. When you saw her after five years, you couldn't help but notice how great she looked. You may have even felt jealous and wondered (even asked): How did she do it?

- You join a new gym. When your fitness instructor walks into class, you immediately evaluate her own fitness level by her size and how toned her body is.

- When your track coach suggested you could drop a bit of weight so you could run faster, you felt her criticism and judgment. But you didn't question it or deny it. Instead, you started to eat only salads for lunch and dinner.

- You would watch your mother get dressed for work, and she would ask, "Does this make me look fat?" You find yourself asking the same question.

- When you received your raise at work, you were happy, but part of you thought you would be happier if you had your raise and also lost ten pounds.

So subtly, we've haven't just been receiving these messages. We've also been offering them. Unknowingly, you and I have spread this belief around with our thoughts, words, and energy.

THIN IS SO MUCH MORE AND FAT IS SO MUCH LESS

Our cultural assumptions around thinness reach further than happiness, attraction, and success. Thin women are assumed to be healthier, smarter, fitter, stronger, more disciplined, and richer.

The connection between a thin body and a healthy body can be traced back to the industrial revolution. Later, a 1950s advertisement for the Borg Scale included statements like, "Give somebody a lovely figure for Christmas," "Gladden a heart-slim a figure-with a Borg, this Christmas."[6] More recently, I've heard stories of medical professionals suggesting weight loss to women who are in perfect health.

We hear the message that a thin body is a must to live a happy life not only from the medical community, but also from one of the most powerful places in the world: the White House. Michelle Obama, who's received plenty of attention for her defined biceps, created her First Lady platform called "Let's Move!" According to the program's archived website, "Let's Move! is a comprehensive initiative . . . dedicated to solving the problem of obesity within a generation, so that children born today will grow up healthier and able to pursue their dreams."[7]

Without a thin body, we've been told we're doomed to be unhealthy and miserable.

When Lululemon, a popular retailer for yoga clothing, received criticism for its sheer yoga pants, then CEO Chip Wilson affirmed the thin ideal as he tried to explain his product's deficiency. "Frankly, some women's bodies just don't actually work [for the yoga pants]," Wilson said on Bloomberg TV's Street Smart program. "It's more really about the rubbing through the thighs, how much pressure is there over a period of time, how much they use it."[8]

The gas we've been hearing is so poisonous that when women's bodies aren't thin enough, they are blamed for poor-quality and poorly designed clothing.

Thinness isn't just nice to have. Not being thin means our bodies have been reduced to the lowest of low. Fat means disgusting, despicable, insane, rude, crude. Actually, it's difficult to even put real words to it, as we just understand it as being one of the most feared states.

Just like a thin body brings us the goodness in life, a body that isn't thin is a sentence of shame and despair.

WHAT WE *REALLY* HEAR

We've been valuing ourselves based on our outside appearance, and so has the culture we've been living in. No one has offered us a gas mask to protect ourselves from the messages we've been seeing and hearing. We haven't been judging just our own bodies; we have been judging all women's bodies. We haven't been judging just the physical; we've also been judging the totality of ourselves as a person and the possibility of our future.

The message we've received about the standard of body size has been a personal message. If we can't achieve an ideal body, we can't have an ideal life. Can professional success fully come to a woman who's not ideally thin? Can we go on vacation, feel relaxed and happy showing off our body at the beach, if we aren't thin enough? Can we put on our favorite jeans, ones that may not be considered our "skinny" pair, and enjoy a fun night out with friends?

The answer to these questions around how we enjoy and participate in our lives is about how we value ourselves. We may be believing, "No, I don't deserve it," "My body doesn't measure up," or, "I'm not worthy." **If we aren't thin, we can't enjoy the good things in life.**

Now, we can wake up and notice the gas for the real poison it is. We must recognize these messages and see how they have eroded our sense of self. We've been believing that if we are fat, we are worthless. And we both know this simply isn't true. There is no merit or cause for these messages, and we must swiftly dismiss them.

But we haven't. We've let these messages fuel us into action to lose weight. After all, if our body isn't thin enough, we haven't resigned ourselves to an unhappy life. Like the American dream, we believe in an opportunity to sacrifice and work hard for a better life. If our body isn't thin enough, there is a way for our body to reach the ideals of physical beauty. It's called dieting.

CHAPTER THREE

Diets: Hungry for Happiness

Ninety percent of women are unhappy with their bodies, and now we know why. We've been driven to lose weight, and diets are well understood to be the answer.

If you want to lose weight, go on a diet.

Another statement we believe to be true.

In the 1970s, the average age a girl first went on a diet was fourteen. Now, in 2019, the average age is eight. According to a self-reported survey, half of all Americans are trying to lose weight.[9]

Our need for a thin and lean body has led the government, the weight loss industry, and the health-care industry to seek a way for us to lose weight. The weight loss industry alone is a massive $70 billion industry filled with diets, programs, specialized food and supplements, and medical procedures.

Let's define diets as a prescribed way of eating with rules and guidelines for weight loss. Certain foods are limited and excluded as well as limited on quantity and calories. Measurements of foods like grams of fat, protein, carbohydrates, sugar, or fiber may be increased or decreased depending on the diet. Essentially, when following a diet, there are limits and restrictions.

The Hollywood diet, also known as the grapefruit diet, was introduced in the 1930s for actresses and actors to drop weight quickly. With experts claiming that grapefruit contains an ingredient that promotes fat loss, dieters ate half a grapefruit at each meal for ten days.

Almost a century later, dieting and weight loss isn't just a fad or something that's done only by actors and actresses, the overly health-conscious, or the athletic. You and I have tried countless ways to lose weight—low-fat and high-fat, low-carb and high-carb, no-sugar and all-fruit. There is no shortage of ways to lose weight.

DIETING VS. GETTING HEALTHY

From a young age, weight loss was always on my mind, but I never called it dieting.

Admitting to anyone that I was trying to lose weight would be admitting I was overweight. Sharing my tactics left me open to others' scrutiny. If they hadn't denounced my need to diet, they would have confirmed my worst fear: I was overweight. If they had agreed, then I needed to diet. No, I would keep my weight loss strategies to myself and avoid the risk.

Instead, I claimed I wanted to be healthy. Feel strong. Get lean. I knew which foods to avoid and which ones I could eat more of. I believed I was trying a new lifestyle, creating better habits, something I could do for the rest of my life.

My friends also had their weight loss goals. Colleen, my roommate after college, and I would buy baked low-fat potato chips and diet soda. Debbie and I didn't just go to yoga together; we also went on a ten-day juice cleanse together. And thanks to Amanda, whom I met at a breast-feeding support group, I tried Weight Watchers to lose the extra baby weight from my first pregnancy.

No matter what I called it, trying to lose weight meant I was restricting what I ate and how I ate it. Restricting was something I did, and I did it in good company. But the reality was, anytime I was trying to lose weight, I was dieting.

DIETING TAKES ON DIFFERENT NAMES

In the past decade, "diets" have gotten a bad reputation. Dieters don't want to starve themselves and give up their favorite foods. However, that doesn't mean women don't want to lose weight. They still do. So weight loss products are now being marketed with more complexity. They promise us slightly different results for the same goal. For those women like me, unwilling to confess our weight loss goals, we get enticed with promises to:

- Curb our appetites
- Reduce cravings
- Increase our metabolism
- Improve our ability to burn calories
- Make our fat cells smaller
- Increase our feeling of fullness
- Give us more energy
- Manage our weight

They don't need to promise us weight loss anymore. It's just a given that we want a thinner body. Instead, they help solve all the struggles we have with weight loss without having to even mention the "d" word: *Diet*.

Marketers and diet companies are relentless in how they try to motivate us to persist with their weight loss products. They suggest we don't give up on ourselves ("It's not a diet, it's a lifestyle") and keep sacrificing ("Nothing tastes as good as skinny feels"), and that we can achieve our goals if we just stay focused enough ("Get up every morning and tell yourself, 'I can do this'"). Marketers are geniuses at playing to our desire to improve ourselves and improve our lives. Which, as we know, simply means having a thinner body.

They do their best to convince us that joining their diet will make us a better version of ourselves. They understand our desire to have a better life.

EVERYONE MUST BE ON A DIET

Recently, a Wendy's commercial came on during a football game I was watching. This fast-food giant was advertising its latest chicken sandwich. "Isn't that what a cheat day is for?" it asks. In fact, there is a well-known diet that calls for six days of dieting and one off day—or a "cheat day." By suggesting we can have a cheat day, Wendy's is letting us know we must be dieting.

The need to lose weight with dieting and restriction is another undetected gas. Restricted eating has permeated its way into our culture. If we are all trying to lose weight, we are all doing one thing: dieting. That's why weight loss is discussed widely on social media, in gyms and fitness centers, at neighborhood bus stops, and around the coffee pot in office kitchens.

In our culture, dieting and weight loss is a way of life.

WHAT'S THE PROBLEM HERE?

If the grapefruit diet offered long-term weight loss, there wouldn't have been a need to try another diet. And similarly for you and I. If the rules and guidelines of Overeaters Anonymous had worked for me when I first dieted with my childhood friend, I wouldn't have needed to try a second one. Or third one. Or twentieth one.

At one time we listened to music by painfully creating mixtapes with our Walkmans and cassette tape players. Because the global recorded music industry keeps innovating and delivering solutions that work and fit our needs, we can now listen to, compile, and share our playlists through the convenience of our phones. The same can't be said for weight loss products and diet programs. An already massive industry continues to grow with different solutions that still don't work.

L.L. Bean, an outdoor retail store headquartered in Maine, offers a full money-back guarantee within one year, no questions asked, on everything from their tents and lamps to their flannel pj's. The company stands behind the products to work as intended. I reached out to customer service at both Weight Watchers and Jenny Craig asking them if they offer a guarantee on their products. They both do not.

As consumers of the weight loss industry, we haven't demanded a guarantee or innovation with permanent results. We have been buying its products, crossing our fingers that this time they may finally work, because it's expected of us. We've developed a secret pact with an industry that has done nothing more than taken our money and left us feeling defeated and weighing more than we did before we tried their products. We don't hold them accountable for their claims of weight loss because when we fail, we suspect that we did not follow their program as prescribed.

The reality is, diets and restrictions aren't designed for long-term success.

DIETS DON'T WORK

Science seems to agree that diets just don't work. For example, researchers at UCLA reviewed thirty-one studies of diet effectiveness and concluded that diets aren't a predictor of weight loss, but instead are a predictor of weight gain. Two-thirds of dieters gain the weight they initially lost, and even more in the long term.[10]

In a 2016 study by the National Institutes of Health, thirteen of the fourteen *Biggest Loser* contestants regained the majority or even more of the drastic weight they'd lost when they participated in this wildly popular reality TV series.[11] While on the show, the contestants removed themselves from their day-to-day lives, held the public spotlight, and were incentivized with hundreds of thousands of dollars if they lost the most weight. Yet receiving the advice and coaching from the top fitness experts, nutritionists, and psychologists in the country didn't give them a permanent solution. The whole country cheered them on. I personally was moved to tears as I watched their efforts. Yet these drastic measures didn't work in the long run.

The Biggest Loser ran for seventeen seasons, from 2004 to 2016. As a result of these findings, previous contestants demanded the show be canceled.

RESTRICTED EATING IS
FIGHTING OURSELVES

Essentially, when we diet, we are working against ourselves and how our body is designed. It's like pushing a boulder up a steep mountain. As we keep climbing, the boulder gets heavier and bigger. The stricter the diet, with more rules and requirements, often the heavier the boulder.

Let's look carefully at the dynamics of dieting to understand clearly why dieting and restriction never works for the long term.

We Focus on What's Forbidden

Our minds are pretty remarkable. When we choose to focus on something, the energy around what we give our attention to increases. Have you noticed what happens when you consider buying a new car? Take a Mini Cooper, for example. You notice Minis at the grocery store and in the school parking lot. They are everywhere you look. But there really aren't more of these cars. Instead, your attention has been on them, and so you notice them even more.

When we diet, we need to avoid certain foods—carbs, sugar, processed foods. You know what's on the "bad food" list. By focusing on avoiding a certain food, our energy and momentum increases around that food. Yes, even though we are trying to avoid that food, our brain doesn't distinguish between wanting more or wanting to avoid. It just knows what we are placing our attention on.

It can be difficult to avoid a food we're trying so hard to not eat, as the harder we try to avoid it, the more energy we give it.

We Want What We Can't Have

We value things more when they are in short supply. When we diet, all forbidden and restricted foods are in short supply.

We understand this concept from economic demands around Christmastime, whether it's for Cabbage Patch dolls, the latest iPhone, or other sought-after gifts. Everyone wants one, but there is not enough supply to keep up with the demand from parents who want to make their children happy on Christmas Day. Do prices go up? Absolutely. When items are in short supply, their value goes up.

When it comes to food, we are afraid of missing out, of losing an opportunity to have something for ourselves that we may not get again. **When a food we enjoy is off-limits and not available to us, we want it even more.**

Consider the holidays, when your aunt makes her famous German chocolate cake. She only makes it once a year. Most diets would not permit a slice of this delicious cake. Yet you know that after it's gone, you won't be able to have a slice again until next year. This creates even more importance and urgency to having a slice for yourself.

This scarcity effect is why staying on a diet is so difficult. People want what they value, and when things are in short supply, the value goes up.

We Want to Make Our Own Choices

The primary motivation of every human being is autonomy. We want to make our own choices. We want to have influence over our own life and exercise free will. We really don't want anyone or anything to tell us what to do and how to do it.

When it comes to food, diet plans make our choices for us. Even though we willingly diet for a desired outcome, a strong part of us just wants to eat what we want to eat.

People who struggle to stay on a diet may call themselves rebellious or may even say they are resisting positive change when they go off their diet and eat something they are not supposed to eat. Both are untrue.

There comes a point when we can't stay on our diet any longer. I had given birth to my second child when I joined Weight Watchers for the second time. Once again, I was eager to drop the baby weight like I had the first time I joined. I recalled the diligence, persistence, and commitment I once had and was determined to summon it again. Just a few days into the program, however, I was bored. I would easily forget to log into the tracker and record what I had eaten. I would reach for a scone for breakfast or nibble on chocolate-covered pretzels in the afternoon without thinking twice. I just wanted to eat what I wanted to eat and was tired of following someone else's rules. I was in conflict; my diet goals were confronted by my need to make my own food choices.

We Ignore Our Body's Signals

When following a prescribed eating plan, we weigh, measure, and count all the calories and macronutrients we eat daily. Commonly, diets create a calorie budget based on current weight loss goals and body weight. This formula may also include height and activity level. And it requires strict adherence, no matter our hunger pangs. I remember afternoons when my stomach was grumbling as my body was telling me it was simply hungry. Yet to follow my diet, I had to ignore my hunger.

Dieters know what it's like to distract themselves from hunger. Maybe they chew gum, drink soda or iced coffee, or opt for an allowable snack. Depending on the diet, that could include microwave popcorn, a fat bomb, or carrot sticks.

When we're on a diet, the diet plan is always consulted before the body is. Hunger is generally the enemy, something that can be inconvenient or uncomfortable, as it's an obstacle to weight loss.

Our nutritional needs change with things like age, physical activity, hormone fluctuations, and environmental factors. Yet, diets only offer us predefined standards and measurements and set aside optimal vitality of each individual person. Diets don't account for the uniqueness of each body.

We Feel Guilty

Restricted eating has two partners. They're called repentance and guilt. Often, the tighter we restrict how we eat and the stricter the diet, the more guilt and regret we feel. Like a young child who wants to make his or her parents happy by not breaking the rules, we've been taught that following a diet and the rules that accompany it means we've "been good." When we slip up on a diet, we may not tell ourselves explicitly that we've "been bad." However, we do feel like we've let someone down, done something we shouldn't have, or made a mistake.

When we feel guilty for breaking our rules and restrictions around food, the only way to resolve this guilt is to work harder at following the rules in the future. As you now know, our bodies are not designed to be restricted around food. We restrict, overeat, repent, and restrict. This is how the cycle is created. As long as there are rules to follow that get broken, there will be guilt. And guilt never motivates us to do anything but try to be good and follow the rules. Rules that we simply can't follow. This cycle can't be broken if rules and guilt are both present.

FORMULA FOR SUCCESS DOESN'T APPLY

How we've been successful in some areas of our life doesn't apply to weight loss. I've had my own philosophies around life, ones that guide me when I make decisions. Maybe you can relate to these:

- Keep your head down and just get the work done.
- Stay focused on the goal.
- Put in the extra effort, and you'll be rewarded.
- Do whatever it takes.
- Always have a plan and follow a process.
- Put your best foot forward.
- Be prepared.

These approaches work in school, sports, and professional life by accomplishing structured goals where there is a clear and defined path. And this is why you've been believing that dieting will work for you. Follow the plan, track what you eat, monitor your progress, work hard at it, sacrifice what you can. All diets have been designed to fall into this clear and distinguished structure. Yet as we've discussed, when it comes to the natural way our body wants to be nourished, this approach doesn't work.

CONSULT THE EXPERTS

The diet industry has been convincing us their expertise around nutrition and our bodies is far superior to our own. And with over one thousand different diets and ways to lose weight, the industry has designed schooling, educational programs, and areas of coaching so people can intensively study food and how it works with the body.

Before we dieted, we knew what to eat, when to eat, and how to eat. We've been swept into a culture where food has become so complicated. Does it have to be? Every diet's founder and adherents declare their way to be the optimal way to eat for weight loss, but in reality, our bodies have always known how to eat in a way to nourish ourselves perfectly and maintain our perfect and ideal size.

Diet books have plenty of research backing up their claims on what it takes to lose weight. Even famous entertainers get paid well for promoting and endorsing a program or product, giving us the illusion that if someone we admire tells us to do something, we can trust them.

With every diet we try, we continue to forget and forgo the expertise of our own body and ask someone else to tell us to do something we fundamentally know how to do: eat well.

DIETING REAFFIRMS OUR UNWORTHINESS

Dieting as a way of fixing ourselves and our bodies is like changing a tire on your car when it's not flat. But even worse, fixing the tire will make the tire flat. Without the need to lose weight, we wouldn't need to diet.

Our drive for thinness is a thief and leaves us empty. Thanks to the design of dieting and its inevitable failures, we get to give ourselves this constant reminder. Dieting has been a way of proactively punishing our body, treating it as something that isn't valuable or worthy. Our body isn't thin enough, and neither are we. We don't have what it takes to have the life we want. We can't even lose weight.

Women all around us have reaffirmed this illusion by investing significant time and energy toward weight loss. As you take in the psychology of humans and how that contrasts with diet and restricted food design, use your own dieting experiences as evidence. With a fresh new perspective, consider when your diets failed you.

Along with dieting failure comes the inevitable, "How could I let myself get so out of control?" and, "Why can't I do this?" and, "What's wrong with me?" questions. By answering these questions, we start to feel the personal impact of our dieting. This impact includes labels around our behavior and fears.

Diets simply don't work, and ultimately, they create a long-lasting and devastating impact on the dieter.

CHAPTER FOUR

Labels and Stories: Hungry for Hope

I received my binge-eating disorder diagnosis in my late twenties. I now had a formal diagnosis by the medical community. It was official. This was serious. Someone with a medical degree determined my eating patterns as a disease.

I asked myself, What was I doing wrong? All I was trying to do was lose weight. I just wanted to be thin, lean, and healthy. How did I get to be disordered?

This wasn't the first time I had a name for my eating patterns.

I read Geneen Roth's *Feeding the Hungry Heart: The Experience of Compulsive Eating* in college. My elation was palpable. Yes! Finally! Someone understood me! Geneen let me know there were other women in the country who were also compulsive and doing what I was doing. As I read about Geneen's eating patterns, gaining and losing more than fifty pounds over several months, I felt oddly comforted. I wasn't alone. I was understood.

As a self-declared compulsive eater, I was part of a tribe of other unknown women who also struggled with food like I did. As far as I knew, my friends weren't compulsive eaters. They didn't know me when I binged. They didn't see me when I felt so sick and overfilled that I couldn't stand to be seen. I felt like I was keeping a secret I couldn't possibly share.

So even though I didn't feel alone anymore, I felt isolated. I was in, but I was out, all at the same time.

My therapist was keen to tell me that I had a binge-eating disorder, but she couldn't tell me why I had it or what the treatment was. Like a puzzle piece you try to force into the wrong place, I had an inkling something wasn't quite right. If I had a skin rash, a clinician could tell me I had a virus and give me a prescription. With this diagnosis, I was expecting answers, too. Instead, I just had another name to call myself.

THE POWER OF LABELS

Labels are a natural way we describe our talents, abilities, and strengths. Or lack thereof. My daughter plays basketball. She calls herself a basketball player. I run. I'm a runner. My oldest son doesn't even need to say, "I'm good at math," because his quiet confidence and ability to teach himself even the hardest of concepts is something that sits within him. He owns his own label of how smart he is in math. My youngest son feels the same way in English. This is how he knows himself.

Labels can hold limits and they can also hold possibilities, but the real power comes with which ones we attach ourselves to. When we believe, deeply, that we have talent and skill, we will make choices consistent with those beliefs.

If we believe we don't have a skill or our brains don't work a certain way, we won't take risks, we won't expect solid results, and we won't be part of a group of people who do possess the skills we don't have.

LABELS LIMIT

Now that I had another name to describe my actions, I had no choice but to determine what "binge-eating disordered" meant to me, just like I did with "compulsive eater." I equated them with being out of control, disgusting, and fat. Every binge, every box of cookies, every bag of chips was evidence of both diet failure and of being disordered. After every binge, I now had a label for myself that reminded me of my too-big body. What do compulsive eaters do? They eat. They eat in an out-of-control way. They eat lots of food and gain weight. They're fat. They're broken.

With every label, we create a further complexity to explain why we overeat, or binge, or undereat. Each label makes our relationship with food even more personal and reinforces the poison of the invisible gas we've been subject to. Our body is not good enough. We can't succeed at weight loss. And now, the medical community and other experts have sentenced us to an illness, disease, addiction, and disorder. Whether we do in fact have one or not, the label itself is enough for us to believe we are truly damaged. And we choose to eat in a way that's consistent with these labels we use to describe ourselves.

With my label, I got to create my actions—actions that are consistent with being a compulsive eater and a disordered binge eater.

We are flooded with ways to describe our eating patterns.

- Sugar addict

- Binge-eating disordered

- Compulsive overeater

- Disordered eater

- Carb addict

- Stress eater

- Emotional eater

- Chronic dieter

These labels used to describe our symptoms each hold a subtle distinction to tell us what our problem is and how it will predict our doomed future. What is our weakness? The label answers that question for us. It's sugar. Carbs. Stress. Emotions.

"BIG-BONED" STORY

When I was a young girl, my grandmother called me "big-boned." I didn't quite understand what she meant, so I would wrap my forefinger and thumb around my wrist to measure just how big my bone was. If there were big bones, there must also be small bones, I thought. I would also measure the bones of my cousins so I could compare their bones to my big bones. Grammy didn't call them big-boned. Just me. After much thought and many wrist measurements, I concluded I was heavy, large, and bigger than others. Was I fat? Yes. This was obvious. Big-boned and fat.

Without realizing it, my story around the size of my body was crafted. My mind made assumptions around what "big-boned" meant. And every wrist measurement was my way of gathering more evidence to support these assumptions.

I would compare my jean size with those of my friends. Yes, I was larger than they were. I saw pictures of myself and how large I was. When I ate more food than my cousins, I assumed it must have been because I needed more food than they did. After all, I was bigger than they were.

My big-boned self was not like the bodies of other girls, and eventually women my age. I was different, too big, too much. With the messages I had heard around how we value thin bodies in our culture, I also believed I was fat and disgusting.

I didn't know this was a story I had created in my mind at the time. This is just how I understood myself and the world. It just made sense to me. But as I started to become aware of my own beliefs around my body and understand where they came from, I realized I had been telling myself a painful story.

It's amazing, isn't it? So complex. How one small statement from my beloved grandmother could morph into something so personal and painful. Stories have that power, especially when fear is fueling them. Two words, casually tossed out, can be interpreted as a threat to feeling loved and accepted. Two words have the power to make us believe we aren't good enough.

WHAT STORIES ARE

Along with the labels we own, we've also created stories. Stories are narratives we create in our minds as a result of our fears. Stories bring life to our fears and make them appear even more real. It's our stories, when we've connected the dots between one thing happening and an expected outcome, that tell us how we can keep ourselves safe.

Fear is a response to a perceived threat. One type of fearful response can be primal and automatic. When our toddler starts to run into a busy traffic street, primal fear automatically puts us on high alert and drives us to action to bring them safely to the sidewalk. Primal fear is critical to protecting us and those we love. Thankfully, this kind of fear is rare.

We are more familiar with the second type of fear— fear as an emotional response to a perceived threat. I was only ten or so when I'd be woken up in the middle of the night by a tapping on my bedroom window. I'd be so scared that I'd lie there frozen, clenching my blanket for safety. My friend had recently told me a believable and scary ghost story, and I was convinced that tapping was a ghost. My fear of ghosts was an emotional fear.

Every human being wants to feel safe, loved, and accepted. This is why we fear rejection, we fear being alone, we fear being judged, and we fear failure. Our basic human desires need protecting, and fear is masterful at trying to protect us from anything that may threaten us.

Stories are our way of gathering evidence that our fears are legitimate. Both types of fears are designed to keep us safe. One, from a very real and tangible threat. The other, from a perceived threat. Our body doesn't distinguish between primal and emotional fear. It reacts in a similar way.

When we experience fear, we feel it in our body. The fight-or-flight part of our brain, the parasympathetic nervous system, releases adrenaline, and blood flow to our major organs starts increasing. Our heart rate also increases, our hands can get sweaty, our pupils often dilate to improve focus, and we may feel pressure in our chest. Fear, even from a perceived threat, feels real.

When I heard a tapping on my window as a young child, my safety was in question. Not in reality, but in my mind. (Not surprisingly, the tapping came from a tree branch brushing up against my house when the wind picked up. No ghost. Just the rustling of the tree.) But fear creates stories.

The problem is stories are hard to identify as fear-based beliefs designed for our protection. Our emotional fear feels very real, and it tries to hide itself.

DON'T SEE ME

We've each created our own fear-based story. Like a record player, it just keeps running over and over. Inside each story holds beliefs about who we are, how loved we feel, and how valued we are. Inside these stories we've been telling ourselves our bodies aren't good enough or thin enough.

I met Tracy at a workshop. Charismatic and clear, Tracy was in the business of working with women entrepreneurs. As part of growing her business, she often spoke at events. She described her need to hide when in front of dozens or hundreds of people. "I immediately look for the podium and stay behind it my whole talk," she shared. It didn't take long for Tracy to understand why she hid. Her mind quickly flashed to her days on the elementary school playground, when sports teams were picked. "I was always picked last," she said, tears starting to make their way out of her eyes. Her pain of not being wanted and feeling like she wasn't good enough to be on a sports team felt as fresh as if it had happened the day before. But it hadn't. It had been decades, yet Tracy carried around her fearful story, adapted to situations like public speaking and being on camera, and continued to feel the threat that she wasn't loved and didn't belong. Our fear of judgment and criticism is enough to always want to hide ourselves. **We**

cover our bodies with clothes that are too big or too dark hoping that others won't notice us.

Whether we were bullied on the playground or have experienced violence and abuse, our fear of being seen has been vital to our safety. We may hide in our clothes or put extra weight on our body so we can be invisible and go unnoticed.

DON'T LOSE CONTROL

When Diane and I started working together, she shared her concern about her feelings. Her childhood was really tough, and when her father passed away a few years ago, she had a panic attack a few months later. "I'm afraid of what will get unearthed," she told me. Diane's emotions were unpredictable, and she was afraid of what would happen to her when she felt them. Feeling them meant she may not be able to control what would happen to her. This was Diane's story.

We all have had heartbreak and sadness in our lives, and a common reaction is wanting to put the pain in the past and try to forget about it. Diane's beliefs around not feeling safe to feel her emotions is a common narrative among the clients I work with. Staying in control of how we feel means we don't feel. And it's easier to run away from how we feel. It's easier, for example, to turn to your work or your to-do list and keep busy with those things you know you control.

If we fear losing control and feeling too much, food can be the answer to our fears. Eating and overfilling our body gives us enough distraction.

As I started transforming my own relationship with food, I didn't notice what I was feeling but instead how often I wanted to overfill my body with food. Whether it was a snack or meal, I always wanted another scoop or serving. The extra food made my body feel a little heavier. If I had been floating and feeling insecure, another serving of pasta or another half sandwich brought me down to earth.

When uncomfortable feelings start to arise, food offers us safety in our body. Eating offers us a way to feel secure.

STORIES AND DIETING

Dieters diet because the extra weight on our body is a perceived threat. The message that thin women have it all has created fear in us. By not looking a certain way, we are afraid of not fitting in. In our minds, if we could control what we ate and how we ate it, we would lose weight and finally feel a sense of belonging, love, and acceptance. This is a narrative that's common for dieters to create.

Here are four parts of that narrative we've come to believe.

Don't listen to your body; it can't be trusted. Dieting can make us afraid of feeling hungry. After years of dieting and subjecting ourselves to food deprivation, feeling hungry has been an uncomfortable and unwelcomed sensation. We've learned to stop listening to our body. We've ignored our empty and growling belly. We've dismissed our lack of energy from not having enough food fuel. Some clients I've worked with have eaten defensively, meaning they eat more now in anticipation of hunger, worried they will get hungry sometime in the future. Diets and the volatility of hunger and fullness has given them a version of PTSD; they have a leftover bad memory of being hungry and don't want to experience it again.

You must be perfect. Dieting demands perfection. Following a diet perfectly means we don't take one wrong bite of food. Being perfect is our way of avoiding criticism and judgment of others, but the reality is, in our drive to be perfect, our own critical voice just gets bigger and bigger. The mechanism of dieting is our way of responding to our fears; if we can just be perfect, we will protect ourselves. But instead, a perfect day of eating is often never achieved, and we are left with a voice that tells us we aren't disciplined enough or that we are disgusted with ourselves for slipping up.

You don't have to feel alone. When we are afraid to be alone, dieting gives us community to be a part of. Fear wants to be proven right, and surrounding ourselves with like-minded people is the way we do that. In addition, our fear of being alone and separate will drive us to the security of other people. Being alone and trying to lose weight feels worse for many than it does to try to lose weight in good company. That's why dieting is often done in community. Consider Weight Watchers meetings and online support groups. The diet industry understands the power of community and offers us a way to feel like we are in good company.

You can prove your worth by "winning" at dieting. The dieting industry creatively incentivizes dieters by having them compete for success. Many people by nature are competitive, want to win, and want the accolades and spotlight of success. The Biggest Loser competition is a great example of this, where contestants compete for hundreds of thousands of dollars to prove their success. In the end, someone wins and demonstrates they are better at weight loss than the others. Grassroots biggest loser competitions have made their way to CrossFit boxes, gyms, and even yoga studios. Fear just loves this. Our anxiety around not being good enough can be fed with proving to others in a competition that we can win. And whether we win a free month of a gym membership or we get our picture posted on our gym's social media feed, we are being motivated to prove ourselves.

BRINGING OUR FEARS INTO THE LIGHT

Letting go of dieting and restricted eating can be so difficult for women because it means we have to let go of the labels and the stories we have created for ourselves. Chances are, we've all lost weight on a diet at some point in our life. This alone has created a story within us that has us believing that diets are the way to a thinner body. But as you now know, our fears just keep us dieting.

We don't need to be afraid of our fears. Fears are just part of being human. We are all afraid—it's part of who we are and how we've been designed to stay comfortable.

Our fears don't need to drive us or define us.

The most powerful way we can move past our stories and labels is to bring them into the light. Meaning, take a look at them, write them down, say them out loud. When we can bring them out from the darkness, they lose their power. It's only when they stay, creeping where we can't recognize them, that they drive us. Going forward, we will move toward our fears, not run away from them. When we do, we can see that fear for the knocking tree branch that it is. It doesn't need to paralyze us.

Yearning

PART TWO

♥

CHAPTER FIVE

Blame: Hungry to Be Accepted

What you thought to be the problem isn't the problem. You've been thinking that your food issues have come from food, your emotions are causing your emotional eating, and your body is to blame for your body hatred; these things, however, have only created your hunger. Instead, social conditioning and messaging perpetuating the long-accepted idea that thin women have it all have cut deeper than you may have originally considered. And the long-accepted idea that diets and restrictions are the way to weight loss has led us down a path of weight gain, and so much more destruction.

With every diet failure (overeating, binge eating, etc.), we are reminded that a thin body is that much further out of reach. You've been punishing your body for being the way it is. Your body has been so eager to cry, rage, scream, and sob. But you haven't let it. And that's okay. You're getting closer to the truth and waking up to what's been holding you back from nourishing and loving your body—i.e., satisfying your hunger.

Now it's time to look at why these problems are really not a problem at all. They have actually been personal attacks on us. Let's consider what happens when we believe we are the one causing or creating the problem.

JOE FROM THE CAR DEALERSHIP

When I was in my early twenties and fresh out of college, I bought my first car: a Mazda Protegé. I was so proud of the very first thing I owned myself. After a year or so, I noticed the paint on the hood and top of my car had started chipping. I had never seen this before on any of the cars that my parents had driven, so I took it back to the dealer. The manager at the dealership, let's call him Joe, spent the time to look at my car with me. As Joe inspected my car, he asked me questions like, Was I driving mostly on the back roads or on the highway? Where did I typically park my car? Did I park it in places where nuts fell from trees?And before I got into my car, did I ever put my purse or keys on top of it?

Joe finally concluded that the paint was chipping because of the way I was driving, parking, and getting into and out of my car. According to him, I drove behind eighteen-wheeler trucks on the highway that kicked up debris onto the hood of my car. He knew how often women put their purses on the top of the car when unlocking their doors. He suspected I did the same.

For a brief and naive moment, Joe had me believing that the chipping paint on my car was my fault. Then logic kicked in. Why wasn't the paint on all the other cars on the highway chipped like mine was? His answer implied that I was doing something wrong, that I wasn't treating my car the way I was supposed to. Other car owners weren't as neglectful as I was.

BLAME CREATES SHAME

When Joe blamed me for being negligent, explicitly or implicitly, I could feel the heat of shame that made me lower my voice, avoid eye contact, and want to shrink to half my size. This shame, as I stood in it for just a short period of time, made me feel paralyzed because I believed I had carelessly done something wrong.

I'm confident this was Joe's intention. As a young twenty-something, it took a lot of courage on my part to call his bullshit. Thankfully, his implied attack on how and where I drove wasn't something I took too personally. His blame of me didn't cut me to the core.

But when it comes to why we can't lose weight, the attack is personal. And it hurts us so deeply that we couldn't possibly raise our hand and say, "No! Your weight loss program is destructive, and that's why it's not working for me."

Social media offers plenty of subtle ways to create this blame. For example:

"Eat to fuel your body, not to feed your emotions."

"Food is the most abused anxiety drug. Exercise is the most underutilized antidepressant."

"Note to myself: when I eat like crap, I feel like crap."

"You are not hungry, you are just bored. Drink a glass of water and learn the difference."

Just in case you're not taking my word for it, let's look at those things you thought were the problem. And see for yourself.

CHAPTER SIX

Food:
Hungry for Freedom

With over 50 percent of Americans dieting,[12] we've become obsessed with food. Anyone who wants to lose weight knows which foods are forbidden and which are acceptable. There are certain foods we can eat and certain foods we can't.

We see social media memes like:

5 foods you should NEVER eat
9 foods you want to avoid if you want to lose weight
17 healthy foods that are killing your diet
12 bloat inducers

Millions of research dollars are spent determining the link between certain foods and disease. "Superfoods," we are told, may help reduce the risk of certain cancers. Food has now become disproportionately vital. **We are being led to believe that eating certain foods and avoiding others can create a life-or-death situation.**

I know my body feels differently depending on what kinds of foods I eat. The problem is, when we are eating for weight loss, the power of food has been blown out of proportion. We can't even look at an avocado, a bowl of ice cream, or a slice of bacon without considering its weight loss and health benefits. Or lack thereof.

WE ARE WHAT WE EAT

Jean Anthelme Brillat-Savarin, a French attorney and politician in the early 1800s, wrote, "Tell me what you eat, and I will tell you what you are."

Over time, this notion made its way to the United States and became, "You are what you eat."

A popular meme on social media is: "You are what you eat. Don't be fast, cheap, or easy." We also know fast, cheap, and easy as common ways to describe women who freely offer sex. So, eating a McDonald's hamburger is now equated with being "impure" and irresponsible. Some popular diets, such as "clean eating" and "Whole30," speak to the pureness of the food and the purity of the dieter.

When I was a new mom, I heard some good advice. If your child does something you don't like, let them know that they aren't bad—it was their behavior that was unacceptable. If your son drew a smiley face with a rock on your car's driver-side door, he wasn't bad; only what he did was bad. In other words, don't condemn the person, just the action. We've lost sight of this fundamental truth.

When it comes to eating forbidden foods, people feel good or bad according to how acceptable or unacceptable the food is. Generally, salads fit into all diet plans. When we eat them, we feel accomplished, positive, maybe even righteous. Generally, ice cream sundaes don't fit into most diet plans. When we eat them, we feel rebellious, guilty, maybe even ashamed.

Based on these messages and the education we've received about food, food gives us a way to feel positive or negative things about ourselves. We can feel clean. We can feel pure. Or we can feel dirty. We can feel gross. We can feel fat. We can feel bloated. We can feel disgusting. Food isn't just food, and eating certain foods and adhering to certain diets defines us.

FOOD HAS TO BE AVOIDED

A very well known self-help guru discussed in one of his books how excuses can get in the way of success. He suggested doing whatever it takes to avoid what we should be avoiding. When it comes to staying on our diets, his recommendation was changing our driving route to minimize any temptation that food may have on us.

I know it wasn't his intention, but I immediately felt frustrated by his suggestion. If we've felt out of control around food, it's common to assume we need to extract that food from our lives. Most diet plans and fitness and weight loss coaches also offer the same recommendation. Don't tempt yourself. Take the sugar out of your food pantries, remove the cookie dough from your fridge, and never even pass through the cookie and chip aisles at the grocery store.

But unlike smoking, gambling, or drugs, eating is something we can't avoid.

I heard a similar message at the Overeaters Anonymous meetings I attended. The very first step is to admit that you are powerless over food and your life has become unmanageable. In OA, certain foods are addictive, just like drugs and alcohol.

This is why we believe a cupcake reduces us to our knees and a bar of chocolate can spiral our lives out of control. We need to put energy and effort into staying away from those forbidden foods.

Working a twelve-step program has benefited millions of people and the friends and families who love them. However, if we believe we are addicted, we sure are. If we believe we are powerless, we've forgotten one important thing: every choice we make is our choice and our choice only. No matter what our circumstances are or what conditions we are under, we get to choose what we believe. And we get to choose what we eat and when we eat it.

FOOD IS THE ENEMY

If food is the enemy, consider how we get ready for battle. Several years ago, I remember how excited I was for a night out with my husband to celebrate our wedding anniversary. With two infant boys at home, we didn't get out much. But there was one problem about our date— the bread basket. I wanted to be good and make great choices, but I knew the restaurant we had a reservation at made its own bread, and it was mouthwatering and delicious. I wanted to enjoy my meal with my husband, but I was afraid of blowing it. So, five days before our date night, I was planning how to avoid the bread basket. I kept rehearsing what I would say to the waiter when he casually tried to deliver the basket to our table: "No, thank you, we don't need that; you can send it back."

On our way to the restaurant, I shared my carefully crafted plan with my husband. I was crossing my fingers he would agree. Maybe he would even talk to the waiter for me! But, no, he wanted nothing to do with my plan. He likes bread and loved their bread basket (of course he did) and wanted to enjoy it.

By making the bread basket the enemy, I also made the restaurant, the waiter, and my husband the bread-basket accomplices. It took me so much time and energy to fight against a slice of flour and yeast.

I'm suspecting you've done the same. Avoided the office kitchen when Jim from accounting brought in bagels on Friday. Tried to distract yourself from the receptionist's candy bowl. Ate a "sensible" meal before attending a party or gathering when you knew they wouldn't have diet-friendly food there.

Our tactics have been clever. And exhausting. We've been engaging in a one-sided fight, fighting something that we believe is fighting us back.

WHAT IF FOOD COULD JUST BE FOOD

On the other hand, we've associated so much pleasure and celebration around eating. We share and prepare feasts at holidays and celebrations, cake at weddings and graduations. We also make homemade meals and share them with neighbors who may be recovering from surgery or mourning the loss of a loved one. Promotions and birthdays are celebrated with a fancy dinner out.

In a recent Hershey's chocolate bar commercial, a mother on one side of a bedroom door says to her daughter on the other side, "I know it's hard, Maddie, but I promise it's going to get better," and she slips a miniature chocolate bar under the door. Her daughter opens the door and hugs her mother.

As a mother, I knew Maddie's mom's hopelessness and worry over her daughter's heartbreak and sadness. Thanks to this commercial, I now had a way to solve that problem. Chocolate. It can bring us together and make everything better. The mom said it herself. We receive countless messages like this one that tell us food can comfort us, unite friends and family, and bring us happiness.

Food can be extremely polarizing for those who want to lose weight. On one hand, many foods are forbidden. On the other hand, eating is at the center of community, connection, and comfort. Worlds collide when a dieter wants to be part of this celebration yet can't fully participate because she has to pass on the cake, has to bring her own homemade meals, or, worse, feels so guilty for eating those foods when among family and friends who are celebrating. **Our culture tells us food is how we celebrate, yet the weight loss community doesn't permit us to be part of these celebrations. We are being punished and excluded for the extra weight on our bodies.**

WHAT IF WE JUST LAID DOWN OUR BATTLE ARMS?

"My problem," Paula said so matter-of-factly, "is that I love food too much. I just love to eat." I hear confessions similar to Paula's from many women I speak with around their relationship with food.

Loving to eat and loving food is seen as a character flaw, even a weakness, for those who want to lose weight and get healthy.

Interestingly, Mr. Brillat-Savarin also wrote:

"The discovery of a new dish confers more happiness on humanity, than the discovery of a new star."

"A dessert without cheese is like a beautiful woman with only one eye."

Mr. Brillat-Savarin and Paula have a lot in common. Both understand the magnificence food can have on our spirit and the opportunity for it to enrich our life. Yet along the way, we've lost sight of this opportunity and instead demonized and idolized what we eat. And done the same for the person doing the eating.

The truth is, food is an opportunity to nourish our bodies at a very deep level. When we aren't forbidding ourselves from something sweet at the bakery or a gooey slice of New York style pizza, we can appreciate deeply how we choose to fuel and fill our bodies. We can enjoy the taste of all foods and spend time preparing meals that we know we will enjoy fully.

We've been depriving ourselves of these pleasures. We've been afraid to love food and love all kinds of food. We have been hungry for the pleasure and satisfaction that food can offer us. Our hunger is for complete joy and the connection that comes from breaking bread with family and not worrying about gluten and the carb count—and instead eating because food is a loving choice for ourselves and our bodies.

Our complex and confusing relationship with food can cause us to deprive ourselves not just of life's simple pleasures but of feeling our emotions, too. If you've ever thought that emotional eating was the source of your problems around food, you may be surprised to find out it's simply not true.

CHAPTER SEVEN

Emotions: Hungry to Feel Okay

I polled several clients and asked when they first heard the term *emotional eating*. I discovered that they heard it either from a Weight Watchers leader or, like me, they couldn't remember. It was just a term they knew that helped them understand why they were overeating.

I saw a chart, maybe a therapist showed it me, or I had read it in a weight loss book, that claimed we want to eat crunchy and salty foods when we are angry and warm and sweet foods when we are sad. When I was trying to understand my own episodes of overeating, this chart seemed to help. It linked trail mix to stress, cheese and crackers to anger, and ice cream to sadness. I now had a tool I could use to dissect my overeating behavior and inform me how I was feeling. Accurate or not.

If my emotions were causing my overeating, I now had something else to blame. It wasn't just the temptation of food, it was how I felt. By far, this was an even bigger and more serious personal attack.

FOODS MAKES US FEEL BETTER

When we eat a sugary food, like a pastry or a cookie, our brain releases dopamine. Dopamine is the "feel-good hormone" that can improve our mood, make us feel better, and increase our motivation. We can physically alter how we feel, from sad to happy, with one bite of cake, spoon of ice cream, or Reese's Peanut Butter Cup.

I shared with you the first binge I had when I was a preteen. As I've reflected back on what drove me to eat so much food, I realized it was simple. I wanted to feel better. Over time, as I repeatedly overate, I formed a pattern in my mind. If I didn't like the way I felt, food, especially salty and sugary treats, could change that. I even found myself eating if I anticipated feeling uncomfortable, like if I knew I had a big project at work due the next morning and needed to stay up late finishing it. The anticipation of stress and overwhelm was enough to drive me to the food pantry.

We've been told our emotions are the reason we've been overeating and why we choose the foods we do. However, that's simply not true.

NOT OKAY TO FEEL

We live in a culture where it's not okay to express our emotions. Our culture tells us it's a sign of weakness if boys cry and a sign of volatility if girls get angry. Growing up, our elders may have showed us how to express how they felt by not expressing emotion at all. Chances are, they said, "I'm fine," got quiet, or tried to hide how they really felt. Vulnerability around expressing emotions hasn't been modeled for us, but instead, we've been shown how to keep our emotions under control and pretend everything is okay.

And they told us:

"You need to calm down."
"Stop crying."
"Go to bed and you'll feel better."
"I'll talk to you when you've stopped crying."

As a result, we also ignore how we feel.

A pivotal time for me on my healing journey was fully feeling my emotions. Instead of pretending I was okay, situations would arise where I was furious, or filled with jealousy or anger—all feelings I thought were inappropriate for me to feel. I didn't want to admit to anyone that I was petty, reactive, or insecure. But I was, and when I let the feelings come up and fully felt them, it was uncomfortable. I would feel the heat, I would scream, or I would cry. At times, I would feel a sharp pain in my chest.

I never ate while feeling my emotions. Instead, I ate to avoid them.

When we are on the verge of something uncomfortable, eating can soothe us and distract us from feeling.

WHAT ARE EMOTIONS?

Emotions are just an energy that wants to move. They're the most beautiful form of expression we have. They show us how we are living in this world and experiencing it.

Like our two-year-old who demands our attention when we are on the phone, our emotions simply want to be recognized. They want us to look them in the eye and fully be with them. We've been brushing them aside or running away from them as fast as we can, but really, our feelings just want us to stop and let them surface.

BLAMING OUR CIRCUMSTANCES

In our minds, our feelings have been the reason for our overeating. If we weren't so stressed, we wouldn't be stress eating. By blaming our feelings for overeating, we have another way of blaming ourselves for our eating behavior. By doing this, we may believe our circumstances are to blame for our overeating. If work wasn't so stressful, we wouldn't be stress eating. If we weren't in the middle of a divorce, we wouldn't feel so scared. If a loved one didn't just pass, we wouldn't be so incredibly sad.

When one of my clients, Jen, heard about emotional eating from her Weight Watchers leader, she felt the relief of understanding why she couldn't eat just one piece of cake but had four instead. Emotional eating explained her overeating problem, yet it didn't stop her from overeating. As a single mom to three young children, her life with an overwhelming house during the week and an empty and lonely one every other weekend felt like an emotional roller coaster. Jen didn't feel safe to fully feel her sadness, and overeating was able to soothe her immediately. But after she binged, Jen felt ashamed and hopeless.

Overeating distracts us when we start feeling uncomfortable and don't want to feel. However, the aftermath of a binge is even more impactful and painful than the feeling we initially may have been avoiding. Wanting to hide when we overeat erodes our confidence. We feel far worse after a binge than we did before. Why? Because we have an achy belly overfilled with food. We may worry we will gain weight. We tell ourselves we are disgusting and out of control. Because of our definition of emotional eating, the only thing we can blame for this behavior is ourselves and how we feel.

Feelings are our savior. They are an energy that wants to move through us. Getting to know them and being with them is simply getting to know ourselves. Feelings are an expression of ourselves. Feeling our feelings takes courage, as doing so sends a deliberate message to ourselves that we are okay. We are okay to be sad, and therefore we will feel sad. We are okay to be angry, and therefore we will be angry. Feeling isn't just about the emotion as much as it is about being okay with ourselves. And being okay with ourselves includes learning to appreciate and respect our bodies.

CHAPTER EIGHT

Your Body: Hungry to Be Seen

The cultural messages of ideal beauty and body size show us only one version of a desirable body. It's a thin one. As a result, 89 percent of women want to change something about their body.[13]

We've internalized these messages and have been putting our bodies under scrutiny. We've turned to our partner or best girlfriend and asked them how we look in a new dress or if we look fat in our new jeans.

BODIES GET MEASURED

Sue kept one scale in the kitchen and one in her bedroom so she could conveniently step on it two, three, sometimes five times a day. Sue knew to always step on the scale first thing in the morning, after she'd gone to the bathroom and before she had a single sip of water. Each time she did, the number she saw was compared to her own expectations. If she had been working out more than usual and just had a salad for lunch, she would hope the number would go down. If she just had cocktails and appetizers the night before with friends from work, she would hold her breath but suspected the number may be higher.

By measuring our weight, we can measure our diet progress. The scale can tell us whether we are on track and doing enough to lose weight. Our bodies have taken on a bigger significance, however, than something to measure on a scale or with our clothing size. We take each measurement personally, and this has the ability to influence how we feel about ourselves.

Sue would see the flashing number that indicated how much her body weighed, and immediately, her mood, how she felt about herself and the food choices she would make at the next meal, would be set in motion. She may be pleasantly surprised. She may be disappointed and feel discouraged. No matter what, the scale became a crystal ball, determining the future.

When our bodies don't measure up to where we think they should be, we feel like we don't, either.

BODIES COMPARED AND CRITICIZED

On the playground in middle school, the boys called me a "brute." I heard their name for me as more than big and strong. I heard ugly and masculine. I knew I was taller and stronger than the other girls, but this name seemed permanent, like these boys had cast a spell on me and I had a body I could never change. I could never be petite or pretty. I would always be a brute.

For decades, I kept this bullying a secret. I was too ashamed to tell anyone. If I had, would they have agreed with those boys? Would they have not disagreed enough for me to believe them?

We don't just measure our own bodies; people around us have also been evaluating them, comparing

them, and criticizing them. When I was in college and told my uncle's friend that I'd be trying out for the cross-country team, he looked me up and down and suggested that I lose weight.

I've heard countless stories from clients and friends how people around them have made similar comments on their bodies. The comments stun us and leave us speechless. Why? Because we think there is something wrong with our body. When someone tells us we could lose weight or that our nose is too big, we believe them. Today, I'd reply to my uncle's friend with a quick-witted remark if he told me I needed to lose weight. I would have also taken his comment for what it was: untrue and cruel.

OUR BODIES, OUR SELVES

We've made our body something to despise. And when we see it as ugly, fat, crooked, big, soft, or otherwise, we see ourselves as ugly, fat, crooked, big, soft, or otherwise. We can't criticize our bodies without criticizing ourselves.

Despising something often means we ignore it, neglect it, or even go out of our way to let it know how much we hate it. And that's how we've been treating our body. Self-care is such a hot topic right now. We are being convinced that taking care of ourselves is so important, yet I hear repeatedly how hard it is for women to take time for themselves. They may be thinking that getting enough sleep is an indulgence. Others' needs come before their own. It's incredibly challenging to get someone to care for something they don't care about.

Consider that ugly sweater you got from your mother-in-law for Christmas six years ago. You wish you could give it to Goodwill, but you would feel guilty getting rid of it. Instead, it's squished at the bottom of a bin in your attic. You see no need to care for it. Just like your body.

I splurged a few years ago and bought myself a gorgeous cashmere wrap. The moment it came in the mail, I loved it even more—its softness, the color, and the weight of it on my body. I love how I feel when I wrap myself in it. Warm, cared for. I take great care of my wrap; that way, I know it takes care of me. I fold it neatly and have a perfect home for it in my closet. After all, something so important to me deserves to be cared for.

Your body is designed to offer you the same warmth and security, expression and love as a cashmere wrap. Like something you feel so grateful for and appreciate, your body wants to be treated with great care and respect.

WHAT OUR BODY REALLY IS

When you can see your body for what it really is, you will see that it's a perfect machine, designed to be balanced in an optimal way. When it's out of balance (or homeostasis), it lets us know. Our body holds the wisdom of hunger and fullness and knows this without negotiation. Our body lets us know what we are feeling as it holds our emotions.

We aren't our bodies—our bodies are beautiful shells that we get to inhabit. We get to live through our body. We aren't our bodies.

Really, our bodies are the only thing we can possess. Our homes, cars, and clothes could be taken from us. but not our body. It's the one thing we can claim. Why wouldn't we want to care for it and cherish it? Our bodies are, in fact, brilliant and worthy of our best care.

Discontent

PART THREE

CHAPTER NINE

A Different Perspective

Now, we know where this emptiness around dieting came from. We've heard messages that our body needs to be thinner, that the solution is to restrict what we eat and how we eat, that labels have been created to help us understand our messed-up relationship with food, and that fear has left us paralyzed.

We can also recognize the longing. We've been making food, our emotions, and our body the enemy. But they aren't; they are an opportunity for us to shift our whole relationship with ourselves—by exploring the pleasures of food instead of forbidding it. By allowing ourselves to be messy and feel our feelings. By seeing our body as a one-time gift and not letting a single day pass without treating it with gratitude.

We've spent time looking at each of these different influences. Now, let's understand clearly how these influences have really impacted our lives, because we haven't been experiencing our relationship with food and our body in a bubble. It's really been pervasive.

To get a completely different perspective, let's take food and dieting and body image and weight loss out of the equation by hearing Julie's story. I made Julie up, and she is also hungry. She lives in a fictitious time and has had an experience similar to ours. Julie doesn't need her body weight to change; Julie is desperate to change the color of her hair.

LET'S HEAR FROM JULIE:

When my mother got ready for work, she'd look in the mirror and frown at her purple hair. She'd ask me which scarf looked best to cover her head. When we watched shows together, she always commented on how beautiful other women were when they had green hair. I often borrowed my mother's scarf, and sometimes wore my own hat, to cover my blue hair too. Just like my mother.

There were some really popular girls at school with green hair. I always noticed the cute boys staring at them. The green-haired girls didn't need to hide their lovely locks, and I don't blame them. They were beautiful.

When I got to college, my roommate told me how she turned her purple hair green. I didn't think it was possible, but I was willing to try. I just had to sleep three hours a night. My roommate was such a big help; we worked together to keep ourselves awake. After twenty-five nights straight, with minimal sleep, my blue hair turned green.

I went home on Thanksgiving break and put away my scarves and hats. My old high school friends kept telling me how great I looked. My mother told me how proud she was of me. Most college freshmen slept more than I did. They called it the Freshman Yellow because their hair faded to yellow with the extra sleep. But not me. I knew what it took to have green hair. Sleep sacrifice was worth it.

I got back to school, and finals really stressed me out. I started stress sleeping, but I couldn't let my roommate know. I would take naps while she was in class. Every time I overslept, I felt so guilty. I was getting worried. What if my green hair went away?

Sadly, when I graduated from college, my hair was a dreaded yellow. The stress sleeping became a really bad habit. I had high hopes, though. With a fresh start at my first real job in a new city, I would turn my life around. I'd do whatever it took to get my green hair back.

Scientists had extensively studied the hormones that produce green hair and found that when the optimal metabolic efficiency (OME) was optimized, these hormones would be produced. A friend at work took me to a dimm. Dimms had a special dark room that helped improve my OME. Now, I could sleep a bit more if I spent more time at the dimm.

I felt so much better going to the dimm. When I wasn't working, I was at the dimm. Sometimes for over two hours a day.

My commitment to the dimm paid off. Sort of. My hair did turn green, but it wasn't green enough. It wasn't like it was when I was a freshman in college. I was trying so hard to reach my goal color. My friends and my mother were so encouraging and were always cheering me on. Yet I just couldn't do it. Achieving vibrant, beautiful green hair was always a bit out of reach.

I watched so many videos from experts on how to improve my OME. They all had different opinions and approaches. Some said sleep in thirty-minute increments over a six-hour period. Some said sleep two hours for three nights and four hours for four nights. It was confusing and frustrating, because no matter how hard I tried, I couldn't follow their plans. I was sleep binging every few days and hated myself for it.

I invested in an OME monitor for home. I like tracking my progress and keep it in my bedroom. I use it right before I go to bed. That way I can get the best reading. When I see good results on the monitor, I feel awesome and know I can stay awake forever. But when the results are bad, I want to throw in the towel and sleep even more.

Between you and me, sleep just makes me happy. I love it when my eyes don't hurt and I have the energy I need throughout my day. Why can't I just sleep like normal green-haired girls? I feel like I'm being punished sometimes.

I found a quiz on a therapist's website called "Do you have a sleep disorder?" I took it and not surprisingly, I do. I saw a new drug advertisement that could reduce my sleep cravings. The side effects include dry mouth, dizziness, vision changes, and irritability. Compared to my bad binge stress sleeps, this is a small price to pay. A therapist and a prescription may be all I need to get my dark green beautiful hair back.

I've decided to try one last thing before I find a therapist. I saw one of my favorite high-profile celebrities on video, and she is now part owner of Sleep Watchers. I just love her, her show, and her book club. She's so inspiring. She's had her own struggles to achieve green hair, and she's definitely someone I can trust. I love that she says Sleep Watchers isn't just about the green hair, it's about being happy. So true. That's what I want. I want to be happy with my dark green hair. The community and accountability with Sleep Watchers is so welcoming and supportive. But I have to admit, it's hard to track every sleeping moment.

Now, I'm a mom and have a beautiful daughter. She was born with gorgeous shiny black hair. Everything about her is perfect. But she wants green hair, too, and I feel torn. Struggling for green hair has been exhausting, but this is just the way life is. This is what I need to do to feel good about myself, and I want her to feel good too.

We decided to work together on optimizing our OME. Nothing drastic. Just slow and steady progress. This is a lifestyle change, something to do for the rest of our lives. I try to model balanced choices, and when there is a special occasion, like Christmas or a birthday, we can treat ourselves and sleep six hours a night. I want my daughter to know that moderation is key.

Some nights, I jolt myself awake after too much sleeping. I wonder why this is so hard. I'm either so tired or so lethargic from oversleeping. I don't know any differently. I can't image just sleeping when I'm tired and waking when I've had enough rest. That's foreign to me. I feel trapped. I don't know of any other options.

IF WE COULD, WE'D TELL JULIE:

Please, sleep! You need to get your rest. Your hair is beautiful. It's okay that it's a different color.

Why are you going to the dimm? It's a waste.

Julie, stop the madness. You don't need to work so hard and spend so much energy trying to change something that doesn't need changing.

Right? **It's easier for us to witness Julie's hunger than it may be to witness our own.**

But the truth is, Julie's pain has been our own pain. We know her guilt, shame, celebration, and mental exhaustion. It all started for us when we didn't believe we were enough the way we were. Julie heard the message that she needed green hair and never once questioned it. We heard the message that we needed to have a smaller body and never once questioned it.

Our mothers heard the messages of ideal beauty and without knowing, they passed them down to us. The only way we wouldn't have heard them would be if they had called out the lies and let us know how wrong those messages were. When the Victoria Secret's Angels paraded down the runway, they would have said, "Your beauty isn't about your body; your beauty is so much more."

Only when Julie saw her own daughter's beautiful black hair did she even consider the absurdity of it all. But even then, she didn't know of any other solution. She was living in a culture so permeated with a solution that didn't work that she knew of no other way out.

Mothers often come to me when they have young daughters and realize that they don't want their beloved to struggle with food and weight loss the way they have. They don't want their daughters to step on the scale and let it dictate their day. They don't want their daughters to go prom-dress shopping in tears because they hate how they look.

Our daughters don't need to be our wake-up call. Let's wake ourselves up for our own sake. We deserve more than to always be sacrificing.

We know how ridiculous it is to limit, control, and monitor our sleep. We know humans need to sleep to function optimally and that being tired is a sign that it's time to rest. The same goes for food. Our bodies know optimally what foods we need and what quantities are required to thrive. Our bodies are designed to act perfectly, requiring basic needs. Sleep and food are meant to energize us, restore us, fuel us.

Julie saw different hair colors. Blue, purple, black, yellow. Yet they weren't enough. She gave up so much sleep so her hair could be green, the ideal, the prettiest, the color she needed to have.

We've been doing the same with our bodies. With one out-of-reach thin ideal, we've been neglecting all the body sizes and shapes that human beings come in. We've been sacrificing our own peace and sanity.

We can easily celebrate hair colors representing a rainbow. It's time to celebrate the rainbow of various sizes of real women's bodies.

CHAPTER TEN

Hunger

Before we work together, I always ask a new client how many hours a day she spends thinking about food, weight loss, and her body. Without fail, her response is "always." When we get more specific, it's between six to eight hours a day. Almost half of our waking hours are consumed, hijacked really, with what we just ate, what we plan to eat, how we will lose weight, what diet we can start, and how we wish our thighs and ass were thinner.

In a given month, that's over two hundred waking hours. In a given year, almost three thousand hours. In a given decade, nearly thirty thousand hours.

With our minds so busy, we've been missing out. These hours have passed us by, and we have lived them preoccupied, worried, uncertain, and separate.

HUNGRY TO RELAX

While in college, I walked through my student union center one afternoon eating my lunch. An apple. That's all I would allow myself. A tall, cute guy came up to me, asked me to sign a petition for him, looked down at my apple, and asked, "Why are you eating an apple core?" His casual comment and obvious observation embarrassed me. He didn't know that this wasn't a snack or an appetizer. It's all my diet would afford me to eat.

I wasn't ready to part with lunch. Not yet, anyway. I was determined to find a few more nibbles.

It took so much of my focus to only eat this apple for lunch and ignore my grumbling stomach. What most of my fellow classmates were eating for lunch, and what I was eating, were so different. But more importantly, my time and energy were consumed with food. I worried what I'd be eating or not eating. They didn't. I was self-conscious about what others thought about my food choices. They were relaxed.

Our weight loss goals set us apart from others, and it takes so much of our time and energy to do so. We bring our own meal to a restaurant, spend an extra hour or so in the gym, or choose not to eat when everyone around us is.

HUNGRY TO ENJOY

When I joined Weight Watchers a few months after my first son was born, I spent hours on my laptop, logging in my meals and reading through the Weight Watchers blog. I took the time to make big batches of veggie soup and wrote about my goals and monitored my progress in my journal. I had returned to work part-time in my corporate finance job.

I was so worried I wouldn't fit back into my pre-pregnancy clothes that I was determined to lose weight. There I was, a new mom. I was still nursing and pumping in the office. My work responsibilities were the same, despite my reduced work schedule. I was trying to survive on only a few hours of sleep a night. Yet with all these demands, weight loss was my priority. My way of being happy.

I know now that I wouldn't let myself fully experience these uncertain times. I had to keep busy and work toward something I was determined to succeed at. I was scared to fail at work. I was unsure about being a new mother. But I could try to control how much I ate by using my Points budget. Weight Watchers was a perfect distraction.

Meeting our weight loss goals has been a way to control uncontrollable situations in our lives, the times that have been uncertain and unsteady, like being engaged, having a baby, or starting a new job. We've turned our attention away from moments that require us to fully engage in life and focus on controlling an outcome—like dieting and restricting.

HUNGRY TO BE ENOUGH

In the past year, my friend Rose tripled the size of her business and published her first book. Years of dedication were finally paying off. Yet as she reflected on her latest success, she could only focus on how she still hadn't lost those last ten pounds.

She had gone vegan and cleansed. The weight came off for a few months, but then it came back.

She had signed new contracts, landed a paid speaking gig, and had a packed schedule. Yet for Rose, it wasn't enough.

Weight loss needed to be the final accomplishment that would validate the rest of her professional success. We know the belief that has been instilled in us that thin women are more successful. On the other side of this belief is that when we become successful, we can't fully embrace it if we aren't thin.

We may feel undeserving, a fake, and that somehow good things came along only by accident. We never celebrate our successes or pat ourselves on the back for a job well done. Our efforts aren't ever quite acknowledged or rewarded. Because we aren't thin enough.

We can't separate dieting and our body weight from other areas of our lives. No matter what, if we aren't dieting well, we aren't doing the rest of our life well. No matter what raise we receive, promotion we get, or how well our relationships are going—whatever we do, our dieting success and our body weight determines how we feel about ourselves. And it's never enough.

HUNGRY TO BELONG

When I started teaching yoga, I felt like I was part of a club that I didn't belong to. On the cover of *Yoga Journal*, the Lululemon models, even my own teachers and mentors, were fit and lean and had tiny bodies.

I didn't see my body like theirs. I believed if I couldn't look like them, I could at least act like them. I juiced, smoothied, cleansed, fasted, and took meat out of my diet. Yet no matter how much yoga I practiced, how long I meditated, or how many trainings I attended, I felt like I didn't fit because my body didn't fit.

When I opened my yoga studio a few years later, being the front and center of my own business was challenging because I was so self-conscious. I wouldn't teach my own workshops; instead, I would invite teachers from other areas to teach them. I didn't like sharing pictures of myself or putting my body out there for everyone to see.

In reality, when we feel like our body isn't acceptable, we won't let it fit in with any community or group of people. We keep our bodies and ourselves on the outside, not fully engaging in places we don't feel we belong. This is the reason why some of my clients have a hard time joining a gym or practicing yoga at a studio. It's like having one foot in and one foot out, never feeling fully accepted. Only because we haven't fully accepted ourselves.

When I was a brand-new mom and a yoga studio owner, my relationship with food and my body creeped massively into every other area of my life. We don't just diet, we try to control. We can't celebrate, and we can't just let ourselves experience the crazy yet precious times in our life. It's important for you to take an honest stock of this for yourself. Time is precious and not something we get back once it's passed. You get to have a say in how you spend your time and energy, and now, you can choose differently.

Your true hunger has been this deeply personal longing, a hunger that everyone holds. As human beings, we are wired to want to be seen in our community, to know our value, and to feel peaceful and happy in our day-to-day life. It's important for you to know this, because you aren't unusual, high maintenance, needy, or asking for too much. Thank goodness. Your true desires are natural and expected. Now, let's understand what's been getting in the way of meeting these true desires. After all, we are here to shift your relationship with food and your body. It's time to create a new framework around how you've been eating.

CHAPTER ELEVEN

Disconnected Eating

How we've been describing our relationship with food is disempowering and destructive.

Overeating, emotional eating, binging, disordered eating, and compulsive overeating. Clean eating, juicing, fasting, dieting. Stuffing, starving. Addicted.

Each of these actions holds its own meaning and stigma around who we are if we eat in this way. If we are on a Whole30 diet, we are clean of the impurities from sugar and don't waste our calories on insufficient carbs. Juicing may remind us of people who have cured themselves from cancer and who believe fruits and vegetables hold superpowers. Overeating is synonymous with fast food and being overweight, overstuffed, out of control, and undisciplined.

We understand the power of labels from chapter 4. Owning the label of "sugar addict" helps us define our actions as someone addicted to sugar. When it comes to our relationship with food, labels have only limited us and robbed us of a future with new possibilities.

The infrastructure that has defined these terms is based on the belief that our bodies are valued only if they are thin. That we as human beings are valued only if we are thin. The infrastructure we've been operating in regarding our relationship with food has been designed to understand one problem:

How do we lose weight so our bodies are valued?

By defining our relationship with these existing terms, we continue to solidify this belief. We continue to affirm a problem that isn't a problem.

Our value as women has nothing to do with our bodies.

THE POWER OF LANGUAGE

Our reality is shaped by our conversations. Our minds are extremely suggestive and readily take in the headlines, comments, and statements we hear.

I recently sat in a women's networking breakfast, and we were all having a group conversation about how to help each other promote our businesses. One woman announced, "Women are terrible at asking for help." She stated her own view, her personal belief. The words were offered as an opinion, yet they could shape the minds of the receiver. Each of us either dismissed it, took it in to consider later, or simply believed it. Her words went through the filters in the room without us really stopping to process whether what she said was true or not.

Imagine if in the same conversation a woman had said instead, "Women do an amazing job asking for help." The opposing opinion, yet a drastically different impact on the recipient.

It doesn't matter what was said, just that it was. Words put a stake in the ground so listeners take in the words and all the meaning the words hold.

One offhand statement will not likely have a significant

impact on the beliefs and actions of each person who heard it. However, the repeated conversations, spoken from the lips of our parents, friends, teachers, news reporters, actors, podcast hosts, and Instagram influencers, among so many others, have the power to change what we believe. It doesn't matter if the words are fact or opinion. Our minds aren't fact-finding machines; they are sponges that soak in what we don't filter out.

Our relationship with food and our bodies has been shaped by the conversations happening around us and through us. We understand this now with the statement, "Thin women are happy, attractive, and successful." For those who believe this, or don't dispute it, the conversation continues to spread through our culture every chance it gets. You and I have also now awakened to the false statement of, "To lose weight, you must go on a diet," and we know how destructive this belief is. Yet we see pictures, statements, and conversations everywhere that support this belief and make it difficult to escape.

SOLVING THE WRONG PROBLEM

If our goal is weight loss, overeating and emotional eating are seen as obstacles, things that stand between our current body and our desired thinner body.

However, if you were to set aside the desire for weight loss, terms like "overeating," "emotional eating," and "binging" simply describe how we eat. We eat more than our body needs. We eat for comfort. We eat large amounts of food. You could be overeating with a single baby carrot, or comforting yourself with a small square of dark chocolate, or eating a lot with a half bag of microwave popcorn. These terms pack a punch only because they assume weight gain.

Julie, our friend from chapter 9, had a sleeping problem. She overslept. Binge slept. She had a sleep disorder. These were problems only because the lack of sleep promised her green hair. Absurd, I know. Julie had a problem only because less sleep gave her a desired result. Without the need for green hair, Julie wouldn't need to change how she slept.

Validating these terms is essentially validating a problem that doesn't need to exist.

THE NEW FRAMEWORK: DISCONNECTED EATING

The real problem that needs solving is we've been disconnected from our bodies. I call this *disconnected eating*. Disconnected eating occurs when we prioritize outside guidelines, rules, and advice from those who tell us how to lose weight over the sensations and experiences we receive from our own body.

When we experience disconnected eating, our quest of weight loss, dieting, and avoiding our feelings has severed our connection to our bodies. We've numbed ourselves to the one source that can guide us on how to nourish and love ourselves.

Engaging in disconnected eating has us turn away from our own bodies and toward the expert nutritionists, doctors, fitness professionals, coaches, and even yoga teachers to be the authority on how we should feed ourselves.

One of my yoga teachers created a personal transformational program through yoga, meditation, and self-reflection. It also included a diet component. For three days out of the forty-day program, participants were asked to eat just fruit. Determined to follow the program as it was designed, I never questioned whether eating this way would be good for me and my body. I followed his advice and expertise. For three days I was exhausted and cranky. But worse were the days that followed. I backlashed from not being able to eat more than just fruit. After the cleanse, my body couldn't get enough. And I ate, and ate—a clear sign that my body didn't appreciate three days of eating just fruit. Ironic, isn't it? A yoga program built on the foundation of connecting mind, body, and spirit offered me a way to completely disconnect from my body. My body gave me plenty of symptoms and signs that it wasn't happy. When my body was retaliating afterward, I know now it was trying to correct itself. It's like my body was asking, Why can't we work together so I can have the nourishment I need to feel good?

With disconnected eating, food may be a way of avoiding feeling the sensations in your body. Humans are emotional beings. In ancient yoga tradition, our bodies are understood to have five koshas, or sheaths. On the outer layer, we have our physical body. As we travel inward, we have the energy body, which holds our life force, or prana; our mental body, which holds our thoughts and emotions; then, our wisdom body; and finally, our bliss body. All these layers are working together, designed to be in perfect concert and connection. Understanding the energy of our body gives us an appreciation for not just the physical perfection of it but also the intrinsic beauty that it holds. Our emotions don't come from our heads, but instead reside within us on an energetic level. Our emotions will always need our attention.

Being disconnected from our body has been the real problem we've been struggling with. **Our body has to have a seat at the table, and we've been kicking it out of the room.** Our body is an infinite source of wisdom, holding for us cues of hunger and fullness, emotion and intuition. Our body is a perfect organism, designed to be in a state of balance at all times. It holds for us emotion, sensation, and intuition.

Disconnected eating comes from prioritizing outside information and dismissing the true intuition and sensation from our body. When we blindly follow the expertise of others, we are essentially shifting the responsibility of our own health and well-being into the hands of someone else. When we acknowledge our own wisdom, we are essentially taking full responsibility for our own health, life, and happiness.

We've been hungry for a different way of living, a different relationship with food, and a new way to view our body. Ultimately, our hunger comes from one missing component: connection. Our disconnected eating has disconnected us from ourselves. When we practice connection, we will no longer be searching for something we don't need. We will see we already have everything we need.

Before we understand what it looks like to move from disconnected eating to—you guessed it—connected eating, let's understand what the journey may be like for you.

It's a vitally important journey and I know you're ready to take it.

Journey

PART FOUR

CHAPTER TWELVE

Crossing the Bridge

You're at a pivotal point, worthy of a pause in our conversation. We've taken the time to completely reframe how you've been thinking about food, your body, and your belief that you need to lose weight. You know now that we won't be solving the problem you thought you had. Like any journey you're about to take, it's important to prepare yourself. Let's make sure you have what you need when you pack your bag.

THERE IS NO TURNING BACK

At this point, you know too much. You can't watch a Weight Watchers commercial the same way—not without hearing the real deception behind the false promises. You can't reread one of the diet books on your bookshelf and follow along like you did when you first got it. And even though you still may be looking in a mirror and not liking what's reflected back, deep down you know that your body would be grateful if you stopped hating it.

When you watch a movie with a dramatic and surprise ending, like *The Sixth Sense* or *A Star Is Born,* you can't take back what you know. In the same way, you can't go back to your old thoughts and behaviors now that you know the real reason why you've been struggling with food and hating on your body.

UNCHARTED TERRITORY

Part of me wants to say I'm sorry. Why? You'll need to leave the comfort and security of what you've known for most of your life. The overeating and undereating patterns. The guilt and shame. Hiding the empty cookie packages and going to bed with an overfilled belly. Even though all of that has been painful, it's familiar. And it's human nature to be comforted by the familiar—even if the familiar sucks. Remember when we talked about fear in chapter 4? When we are afraid, we like things to be predictable.

Stepping forward means you'll be in uncharted territory. It will feel foreign and scary. Not knowing what comes next is a beautiful sign that you are on the right path. And for that, I'm not sorry. After all, you know disconnected eating with so much precision and accuracy. It's dependable and reliable. On this new path, you won't be needing those old patterns, as you will be practicing how to find dependability and reliability within yourself, someone you can depend on.

You won't be going to places that require hurtful outcomes, where you feel worse about yourself, where your sense of self feels defeated. Instead, this path forward is all about working with yourself. You won't need to be afraid of exploring what's on the inside, because no matter what it looks like, it's not broken or damaged. It's just a part of you.

YOU HAVE WHAT YOU NEED

When Dorothy wanted to get back to Kansas, Glinda, the good witch, told her, "You've always had the power to go back to Kansas. . . . [she] had to learn it for [her]self." You will be following your own yellow brick road to learn that you already have exactly what you need.

That's the genius of your path forward. We are packing your backpack with awareness, but you won't be requiring anyone's expertise, program, or protocol. You've been living your life inside your body (you've just been disconnected from it at times). Your body holds the expertise and wisdom you need. Throughout this process, you'll be calling upon it, listening to it, co-creating with it, and ultimately, trusting it.

At one point, we recognized our body's wisdom. We were born knowing our hunger, our thirst. We knew when we were cold, and we knew when we were tired and needed to sleep. Our bodies are so beautifully designed with the utmost genius. They still give us feedback all the time. Going forward, you will be revitalizing your connection to it's genius.

RESPONSIBILITY

You've been feeling the blame that comes from not being able to successfully and permanently lose weight. You've been feeling the shame that comes from out-of-control eating. And you know the guilt that comes from always feeling like you're making a choice that could be healthier, lower calorie, lower in carbs, or without sugar.

It's nearly impossible to claim ownership of a situation when you feel like you've been contributing to the problem and feel guilt, blame, and shame around it.

Maybe you've been blaming both the diet that has

failed you and yourself for failing the diet. You may be blaming your work schedule for you not having enough time or energy to make the changes you want to make in your life. You may be blaming your gym for not staying open late enough or opening early enough for you to work out there. There are endless people, organizations, and circumstances that can be blamed or faulted.

If you knock a glass of water off the counter and the glass breaks on the floor, there is no need to call yourself clumsy. You don't need to blame someone else for moving the glass to the edge of the counter, where it was easier to knock it off. You don't need to blame the tile floor for being too hard or the glass for not being strong enough to not break.

You don't need to blame yourself for breaking the water glass, but it's all on you to clean it up.

Up until now, you've received messages that you didn't recognize. You've been sold on dieting and swept up in a cultural epidemic that's hard to see clearly. And your stories and labels have tried to keep you safe, but they've just been hurtful and painful. All of that has led you to this place of blame and shame. Which hasn't helped to move you beyond your struggle with food.

With your relationship with food and your body, it's not your fault, and it's also 100 percent your responsibility for changing it.

So, when you've truly let go of the internal criticism, taking full responsibility for where you are right now will feel light and freeing. Recognizing that you get to make choices that influence how you eat, how often you think about food, and how you feel about your body is incredibly powerful. As you step forward, know that each step is yours to take. And that's a really, really, really good thing.

TAKING FEAR ALONG WITH YOU

This journey will feel so freakin' scary at times. Scary enough that you may not realize you're even filled with fear. As you know now, fear is sneaky and likes to live where you can't see it or hear it. Even now, it may be whispering in your ear, "These ideas don't make sense," or, "You just need to lose twenty pounds; let's not make it any more complicated than that," or, "Join Weight Watchers tomorrow." Fear has been a prevalent and obvious force among all of us through this journey, and it's not about to go away.

So, along this journey, we will be taking our fears with us. I know it's counterintuitive. Maybe you've been told you need to be fearless and conquer your fears. That just takes way too much energy. Welcome your fears like a companion who has something valuable to share.

When you hear her whisper, "Just lose the twenty pounds already," you can thank her. In the past, that statement would have been enough to try a new diet. The real fear has been kept in the dark.

But instead, you will be having a conversation with your fear. Ask her, "What is it you want to share with me right now?" Because you know, it's not about the twenty pounds. When you sit with her, she may tell you that she's afraid of failing. She's afraid of trying something new and being disappointed again. She's afraid that this is her last-ditch effort and if this doesn't work, she'll really be damaged. She's afraid she doesn't have what it takes or doesn't have the time to spend on herself.

Exploring your fears is your path to your truth. Bring them along.

GET CURIOUS

Within the connected eating framework, you can start to wipe away all the assumptions, stigmas, and biases that have come along with your current relationship with food. If you were to describe all the components of your relationship with food on a blackboard, you can now take an eraser and wipe the whole board clean.

You are starting fresh. Now, imagine you're in front of this newly cleaned blackboard. As part of your journey, you get to create your relationship with food however you choose to. That's right. You've been living under the expectations and ideals that have been imposed on you up until this point. Now, you can create your relationship with food based on your own expectations and ideals.

To do that, it's important that you get curious. Remember, you're charting new territory; you will be seeing things for the first time. When you make food choices, they are no longer in the framework of good food or bad food. Instead, you can make food choices based on different factors, like the taste, how the food makes your body feel, and how much energy you receive from the food. To notice those things, you need to be interested in discovering these answers for yourself.

By noticing, you will also start to witness the impact these patterns have on how you feel. You can't change a pattern unless you know what that pattern is.

When you are curious, you are open to new experiences and being able to witness yourself anew.

WHAT IT MAY LOOK LIKE

You're leaving behind the need to keep yourself locked up tight, shut down, and shut off. As I've considered my own journey with food and my body, one powerful thing has emerged. Trust. As a result, it was common that:

- I just needed to cry.

- My body was sobbing from a very deep place.

- I had no appetite and couldn't eat another bite.

- I felt so warmed with gratitude, I had to smile.

- My body just wanted to move, sweat, and work out.

- I needed the comfort of a warm bath.

- I was tired, so I laid down to rest.

- I laughed so hard that tears were streaming down my face.

- I knew a big glass of water would make me feel better.

- I let myself be seen, sharing my true story in front of a hundred people.

Vulnerable. Unpredictable. Raw. Real. Personal.

You don't know how your body will respond when you start listening to it. You don't know what emotions it holds that it wants desperately to let go of. Have faith that whatever is in store for you, what's on the other side of disconnected eating, is simply a connection to yourself.

You know you've been hungry for more. This journey won't take you away from yourself. Instead, it will allow you to experience your body, witness your thoughts, be in tune with yourself, and embrace your whole self. No longer will you be fighting to change yourself. Your hunger will be satisfied as you will be seeing yourself exactly as you are, and simply moving into a deeper connection with yourself.

CHAPTER THIRTEEN

Connected Eating

Our connection to our bodies is on a range and moves along a continuum over time. Our connection to our bodies can change day to day and moment to moment. Even now, I notice meals that help me feel centered and in tune. I also notice times I snack and miss out on exactly how my body is feeling because I'm running from one thing to the next. Connected eating is a practice.

CONNECTED EATING DEFINED

When we engage in connected eating, we are in constant conversation with our bodies. It requires us to seek out answers to questions like:

- Am I hungry?
- How am I feeling?
- What do I need to nourish and care for myself?
- What information does my body want to share?

Our body is one of the first places we go to for information on how to care for ourselves because our body is worth listening to. When we are engaging in connected eating, we use our body's signals as a compass for our choices. Cultivating a respect for your body is part of the process. Gratitude, appreciation, and compassion are some of the practices you will take on as you start to see your body in a new way.

By respecting your body, you'll start to see the other factors that impact how your body feels.

It's not just food. Sleep, movement, stillness, play, pleasure, and purpose are all pieces to bring into your life so you can engage in connected eating. These are things that bring your body alive and connect you to your vitality. And in the next chapter, we will start practicing exactly that. But for now, know that the more you listen to your body, the more respect and love you will have for it.

What moves you along the range of disconnected and connected eating is awareness and choice.

When eating, were you aware of your body's signals, and did you choose to eat in a way that supported those signals? Engaging in connected eating or disconnected eating is always a choice we get to make.

Have you ever had a gut instinct about something and ignored it? And then you realized after making a choice that contradicted your instinct that you knew better? Or, you knew you weren't hungry but ate anyway?

We've all done this. Ignored our gut, literally and figuratively. When we notice the signals, we also must notice and acknowledge the source that produced them. Recognizing the choice we make, whether it's a bite of chocolate cake or taking a job way under our pay grade, is the practice of connection. At any given point, we can honor our intuition or ignore it. Our choice.

We are walking around with what we need; it's just a matter of reigniting the spark to create a clear communication pathway.

Connected eating isn't the goal; it's simply the result of your ability and willingness to tune into your body when you are fueling it. There is no good or bad. Defining ourselves as a connected eater or disconnected eater contradicts the definition of connected eating and disconnected eating. Let's not add these terms as labels and risk that they be considered good or bad. You've been eating the best you've known how to, even when it's been in a disconnected way. We won't be beating ourselves up for disconnected eating.

INTENTION

To move into connected eating practices, it's important to create a clear intention for your health and vitality. Up to now, we've been reacting to messages that tell us we need to lose weight. Making weight loss a priority gets in the way of connected eating. We can, however, have a clear intention of how we want to nourish ourselves and why we want to do so.

For example, I joined my husband on a work trip to Chicago, and we went out for a special dinner at a steakhouse. Before we went, I knew how much I wanted to enjoy my dinner, but I also wanted to walk out of the restaurant feeling a light contentment. This intention helped me choose my meal, how much of it I ate (based on my fullness signals), and how much dessert I ate.

Your intentions are your own, and they need to be personal. They can change over time.

As you bring your own clarity into how you want your body to feel, you will start to expand all the other vital health practices needed to connect with yourself, like rest and sleep, creativity and play, hydration, and healing practices. Food is just one way to nourish ourselves.

Being clear with your motivations and intentions allows you to measure your own choices against something that's real. You are no longer evaluating your choices based on a moving target, which has been the desire to measure your worth based on your body weight.

NEW MINDSET

When we engage in disconnected eating, we judge and criticize ourselves and the choices we make. When we move toward connected eating, we practice softness. With connected eating, there is no such thing as a mistake. When we practice connected eating, we don't practice perfection or an all or nothing attitude. We give ourselves room for stumbling, tripping, and even taking a few steps backward. After all, berating yourself for not engaging in connected eating is like scolding a toddler for falling when they are learning to walk. It's cruel.

By opening the communication channels back to your body, you are coming home, back to yourself. You've traveled away from yourself, and now, you are simply inviting yourself back. Do so with welcoming arms and a forgiving spirit.

Allowing yourself to eat foods that at one time were forbidden can be a surprising experience. Foods no longer hold any power over you when you are engaging in connected eating, and therefore, you get to taste them fully and witness with fresh eyes whether you like them like you thought you did.

Peanut butter cups were once on my forbidden list. When I finally allowed myself to eat them, I mean really allowed myself to eat them, without guilt or worry that they were going to make me gain weight, I noticed parts of the candy I hadn't before. I didn't enjoy them nearly as much as I had fantasized.

Now, my treats are consistent with what I like to eat. Without any agenda, we get to understand our true likes and dislikes.

As we engage in connected eating, we start with the idea that there is nothing wrong with how we feel. What can be painful is when we don't witness how we feel. Our emotions simply want to be seen.

Welcoming emotions into my body is a constant practice for me. I remind myself that all feelings are welcome, as they just want to move through my body. My emotions are just looking for an expression, not necessarily an understanding. Emotions don't need negotiating with.

SLOWING DOWN

Moving to connected eating means we will be creating more opportunity and space to be in our bodies. We get to be patient, and when the physical signs aren't there, we may need to sit awhile longer to hear them. Slowing down has been something we've all been craving. Our bodies have been asking this of us, haven't they?

When my kids were young, I loved taking them to the movies. Inevitably, within fifteen minutes, I'd be sound asleep. There is no question I was running on empty, as the moment I took the time to slow down, my body caught up with me and demanded sleep. We've noticed our bodies' exhaustion, and now, it's time to tune into it and honor it. Slowing down is the only answer.

Slowing down means we take the time to taste our food, then notice how it feels in our mouth and how our belly feels while we eat and after we've eaten.

THE RESULT OF CONNECTED
EATING: FREEDOM

By connecting back to your body, how you feel, and what you truly want to experience in your life, you'll be liberating yourself. You'll let the messages, stories, and labels drop away and find a true freedom in your life.

As you practice connected eating, you keep reinforcing the trust you have within yourself. As you practice trust, your connected eating will become a natural habit.

Trusting yourself is opening yourself up to all possibilities, even ones that may surprise you.

You'll be creating your own drumbeat, one that only you can step to. You'll be asking, How do I want to feel in my body? How much time do I want to spend taking care of it? What do I love, what lights me up? As you practice connected eating, your body will share with you its opinion on these questions. You've never asked it before, and now it's time to listen to it and trust what it has to say.

CONNECTED EATING SYSTEM

The Connected Eating System is a practice with principles to incorporate into your life that you'll continue to go back to over and over. It's not linear or a set of steps. Instead, the system is a way to work with yourself and your body. Each principle supports the others, and you may practice one or two more than others.

There is no magic pill or overnight solution when it comes to practicing connected eating. But it is simple and something that you will be able to quickly find more and more confidence in.

The five principles of the Connected Eating System are:

- Awareness
- Clarity
- Choice
- Listening
- Alignment

As I share details about each of these principles in the upcoming chapters, I'll also be sharing some practices for you to start incorporating into your day-to-day life. Some of them will not appear to have anything to do with eating, and others will. That's what makes the Connected Eating System unique. These practices are about connecting you to your body, when you are eating and when you aren't.

CHAPTER FOURTEEN

Awareness

The principle of awareness in the Connected Eating System is essentially waking up to your body, thoughts, and reactions. Did you notice I didn't say awareness is becoming aware of how and what you eat? You know now that when we engage in disconnected eating, how we eat is just a by-product of so much more.

How you engage with your body and those patterns you've developed in doing so have been in place for years or decades, if not most of your life. Under the old infrastructure, you've been focused on things that aren't part of the real problem. With awareness, you will be shifting your focus and attention to the real contributing factors.

Creating awareness requires us to step outside ourselves and be observers. My family and I recently traveled to the United Kingdom. Every city and town we traveled to felt so brand-new. We noticed every detail—street signs, menus, accents, clothing, etc. I'm sure a Scottish family would have the same experience if they traveled to the United States for the first time. As you practice the principle of awareness, it will be like finding that "eye-opening, just arrived in a foreign city" response to something that you know like the back of your hand.

Awareness is always the first step to change.

AWARENESS PRACTICE: INTENTIONAL BREATHING

Intentionally breathing is the simplest and quickest way to connect to our body. Our relationship with food has been a series of knee-jerk reactions or autopilot choices. By connecting with our breath, we will be calming our bodies so we can slow down our decision-making process. When you use the power of your breath, you create space between your thoughts and your actions. In this space, you have an opportunity to witness your choices. You have an opportunity to set the course of your actions instead of mindlessly going through the motions.

Besides offering our body vital oxygen, breathing is widely known to support our nervous system, specifically the parasympathetic nervous system, which keeps our body relaxed. When we are stressed or anxious, our nervous system goes on high alert. Like the game of Operation when we fail to remove a body part, the whole board lights up. This is what happens when our stress drives our body into a fight-or-flight response. Steady nasal breathing, however, stimulates the vagus nerve, which runs along our spinal cord and connects to our organs, and in turn stimulates our organs instead of inhibiting them. Our heart rate slows, and we feel calm because our body is calm.

Intentional breathing can also ground you in your body so you will feel less stressed and more relaxed. We make our best choices when we feel relaxed, centered, and calm.

The simplicity of a breathing tool can elude us. After all, we've been breathing since we were born. Breathing is the universal sign of life. We have access to practicing intentional breathing no matter where we are or what we are doing.

Practice: Box Breathing

Practice the box breath three to five times throughout the day. Do five rounds.

Breathe in to a count of three, hold your full breath for a count of three, breathe out to a count of three, wait to breathe in for a count of three.

Bonus Practice: How were you feeling before you started the box breath? How did you feel after? The change in sensations may be subtle, but notice even the slightest detail.

AWARENESS PRACTICE:
EATING WITH ALL YOUR ATTENTION

These days, we aren't just eating in front of the TV, watching our favorite Netflix show or football game; we are eating our lunch in front of a computer screen, catching up on social media with our breakfast, and watching YouTube videos while snacking in the afternoon. We are constantly in front of the screen because we carry a screen around with us.

When our to-do list is a mile long, we naturally try to find ways to save time. Eating while doing something else can be considered a time-saver. We may be eating in the car, at our desk, or just on the run.

When I worked in an office, I would eat quickly and inevitably finish all the food I had in front of me. No matter what. I wouldn't remember how the food tasted,

Bonus Practice: Ground your body before eating!

Notice the sensations in your body and become aware of how they move when you place your attention on them.

Notice the color or texture of a sensation. This awareness may be something that just pops into your head.

AWARENESS PRACTICE: NOTICING YOUR THOUGHTS

We constantly have a dialogue running through our minds. The thoughts can be as simple as:

I need to remember to get almond milk at the grocery store. Or,

I hate my thighs. Or,

Why did I eat that second piece of chocolate cake?

We don't even notice most thoughts; they pass through our minds without our awareness. Now we will start to notice what we think. After all, our minds are very busy and are having conversations all the time.

Meditation can be practiced in many different ways. I often hear students tell me how awful they are at it. This may be an excuse for why they don't want to sit quietly, but the reality is that unless you've been practicing, sitting still and just doing nothing can be hard.

Practice: Noticing Thought, or Meditating

Start by finding a comfortable place to sit. It's often best to have your hips propped on either a pillow or rolled-up blanket. Sitting on a couch or chair is also fine.

Sit tall and start with a few intentional breaths, in and out of your nose. Then, like a detective eager to find evidence and clues, watch for your thoughts. As each passes, notice it. And then watch for the next one. After you've noticed one thought, let the next one arrive.

Practice this for five minutes every day. The morning tends to be the best time for me; however, some people enjoy a meditation practice before they go to bed. Whatever time of the day works for you, take this time every day.

Bonus Practice: Writing out thoughts like a full stream of consciousness is a powerful exercise. It's like clearing out a clogged pipe, but by putting our thoughts on paper every day, we get to witness them fully. Take the time to write out your thoughts, letting them simply stream from your head to the paper.

When we practice awareness, there is really nothing to measure. I know for me, as a CPA, this shift felt uncomfortable, even annoying. I loved the satisfaction of quantifying something, whether it was my effort, an input, or an output. That was one of the enticing pieces of dieting: I always had something to measure. With the Connected Eating System, we no longer need to assess our progress and measure our results. You'll know your progress, but you can't assign it a number.

Awareness is very much like a muscle. It can be strengthened when practiced over time. The beauty of awareness is that there is no turning back. Once you start to listen to your true self, you can't stop. Once you notice parts of yourself that have been hiding, they won't be hidden any longer. Once you start to wake up, you won't let yourself fall back to sleep.

CHAPTER FIFTEEN

Clarity

You can't change something you don't know exists. Once you do know it exists, you can understand how and why it came to be. Clarity is the next principle, one to practice after you know what you want to change. The principle of clarity is identifying your own drivers and causes behind disconnected eating. We've spent a good deal of time understanding all the possible factors that have led you to engage in disconnected eating. However, your journey to this point has been your own unique one. It's important that you understand what brought you to this particular place.

Chances are, you've been feeling stuck in your disconnected eating patterns. Disconnected eating is a dead end and allows for no personal expansion. Observing yourself under the new lens of the Connected Eating System requires you to dig deep and look at your past, including the beliefs you've held and the pieces that have created these stuck patterns. Be firm yet kind with yourself. You'll start saying things like, "I've never considered it this way," "This is new," or maybe, "Really? How can that be important?"

Skepticism and curiosity will accompany clarity and will indicate that you are doing the work. Keep it up, because gaining this insight is just the start of the momentum you've been looking for.

CLARITY PRACTICE: CONSIDERING YOUR DIETING RULES AND RESTRICTIONS

As I mentioned, dieting and restricting how we eat has been so ingrained in our culture, it's rare to find many people who don't have rules they follow around food choices. Eating with rules and restrictions has been a process of trusting some authority outside yourself. Now, I'm going to ask you to identify these rules you've put in place for yourself. When you do, you will start to see why you may feel either guilty, hopeless, or rebellious.

Rules and restrictions that have come from outside experts and weight loss authorities don't belong in the Connected Eating System. Eating to nourish and care for your body will be your primary focus. Before we can eat this way, however, we need to clear out the old restrictions and rules. Some may be so obvious that you've never considered them to be rules, like, "I shouldn't be eating full-fat ice cream." Or, "I always need to eat breakfast."

Practice: Identifying Your Dieting Rules

Identify and write down your own food rules by answering these questions:

- What are bad foods?
- What is your favorite food? Is it bad or good?

- When is it optimal for you to be eating? What times of day? Should you avoid eating before or after any certain time of day?
- What are the right portion sizes for you to be eating?
- What foods should you never eat?
- What foods should you be eating every day?

Bonus Practice: Now that you have identified your own rules, consider letting them go. There was a period of time that I told myself I shouldn't be eating a lot of fruit. I was cautious when I made a smoothie or wanted a clementine at breakfast. My fruit bowl was sparse with a couple of apples accompanying one lonely onion. I was living with this rule without realizing it. When I started giving myself permission to enjoy the fruit I wanted to eat (whenever I wanted to eat it), I was so appreciative. I was grateful to allow dates, pears, pineapples, and kiwi back into my life with abundance. Wiping the slate clean of your food rules is so freeing.

When you let the food rules go, you have no rules to break and therefore no guilt to feel afterward. **Guilt always follows a broken food rule.** Guilt often drives us to stricter rules and potentially more disconnected eating. In this important practice of letting go, you are breaking this cycle.

With the vast amount of food choices available, having guidelines around what to eat and what not to eat is prudent and, when done from an intuitive and connected place, is a part of the Connected Eating System. In the upcoming chapters, you'll create your guidelines to follow around how you want to eat, and following them will be effortless. These guidelines will align with yourself and your bigger purpose.

CLARITY PRACTICE:
FEELING HUNGER AND FULLNESS

With disconnected eating, we've learned how to ignore our hunger and fullness cues. As part of connected eating, we relearn how to seek out and honor these cues. Because they show up in a variety of ways and can feel different for different people, noticing them for yourself is a powerful step in creating trust for yourself.

Hunger and fullness are biological responses to our bodies' need for food. We are born with an ability to recognize when we need food and when we don't. When I was a new mother, I quickly found out for myself that you can't feed a baby who's not hungry. They won't tolerate it. If they aren't hungry, they turn their head in protest, fuss, or fall asleep. Babies trust their own natural body rhythms, instinctively.

We eat in a disconnected way when we eat with measurement or for emotional soothing and avoidance. We never ask our bodies, Are you hungry?

Your hunger and fullness falls on a continuum. Let's assign a number to it for the sake of simplicity. This continuum was inspired by Dr. Michelle May's book *Am I Hungry?*.

Hunger and fullness falls between 10 being the most extreme fullness and 1 being the most extreme hunger.

- 3 is when you are noticeably hungry and may start to feel uncomfortable.

- 5 is when you feel the most content. Essentially, you are no longer hungry.

- 7 is when you are past full.

Practice: Notice Hunger and Fullness

With each meal and snack you eat over the next two weeks, spend time noticing your eating patterns with this continuum. Before you start to eat, use your three-count breath, bringing your awareness into your body and belly. With the continuum in mind, assign your hunger a number. After you have chosen to stop eating, notice your hunger level once again.

Becoming aware of your patterns is the first step, so initially, there is no reason to try to change those patterns.

In chapter 18, we will practice where to start aligning your eating habits to the optimal place for you on this continuum.

Bonus Practice: Notice your own signals for hunger and fullness. When you are hungry, do you just notice your body, or do you also notice that your mind is distracted? Does your mood change? Do you get headaches?

CLARITY PRACTICE: RECOGNIZING HOW YOU FEEL

As we move toward connected eating, we will practice identifying and moving the energy of each emotion we feel through us. As we've discussed, a root cause of disconnected eating is emotions that aren't acknowledged or processed.

Emotions are a way the body communicates with us. Emotions don't last forever. The more willingness you have to honor what emotions you feel and then feel them, the quicker they may pass through. Acknowledging your feelings isn't a sign of weakness. Initially, it will take awareness and a hefty dose of bravery.

As you move to connected eating, your drive to eat when you are not hungry will be a clear signal that you may be wanting to avoid an emotion. The habit of avoiding how we feel by eating can be so ingrained, we may not even realize we are doing it.

Practice: Noticing Your Feelings

Identifying feelings may be easy for you, or you may not notice them until you want to eat. When you want to eat, become aware of where your body is on the hunger and fullness continuum with a body scan. If you are not hungry for food, it's time to get curious. Be willing to practice noticing your feelings with an agreement that you can always eat if you choose to.

A powerful approach is to set a timer for five minutes and agree that for those five minutes, you will be in your body and experience your feelings. Afterward, you will choose again: either to eat or to continue to be with your emotions.

Assure yourself that you are safely willing to be in your body, experiencing whatever sensations your body wants to share with you.

Take a few deep breaths using the three-count breath so you can start to center yourself in your body.

Scan your body, almost like an explorer coming upon uncharted territory and witnessing it for the first time.

Notice all sensations, and without labeling them with an emotion, simply call them the way you see them. Tension in throat. Heaviness in chest. Clenching in belly. Those are just some examples, but begin to find your own way of identifying and noticing these sensations.

Be inside the sensation. Bringing all your attention to it, you can experience it by welcoming it. Ask it what it needs to move and be expressed. Wait to hear the answers your body wants to share with you. Tears may come to your eyes, you may want to scream, you may want to curl up into a ball with a heavy blanket on you. Let your body, and its wisdom, guide you to share how you can be with your emotions.

There is no right or wrong way; you are just inviting yourself to be with yourself.

<u>Bonus Practice</u>: Journal about your experience of being with your emotions. Did a memory come up for you? Write about it. Did you have some insight into a challenge you are facing? Or did nothing come to your mind but instead the energy moved around? Write about it and describe it in detail.

CLARITY PRACTICE: IDENTIFYING YOUR STORY

We know that we've been living with labels and stories that have reinforced our disconnected eating patterns. We won't be running from these stories but instead moving toward them. They have something to share with us. When we hear them out completely, we will invite in a neglected part of ourselves. Call it our darkness, call it our demons, or call it our shadow. No matter. Being aware of our stories and labels is a powerful practice and a necessary one in the Connected Eating System.

Practice: Identifying Your Story

Get out your pen and your journal, and consider these questions:

- What is your first memory of dieting?
- What was the hope it promised you?

Consider the results of your dieting over a period of time. What do your dieting results say about you? What do they say about your character, your strength, and anything else about yourself?

What is your first painful memory around food? It could have been about how much you ate or what someone said or did about what you were eating. What did you say to yourself about this event? How did you make sense of it?

What is your first painful memory around your body? When did you first experience that your body wasn't acceptable and needed to change?

What have you been doing to fight against these beliefs?

Getting thoughts out of your head and down on paper is an important step. When thoughts stay in your mind, they can act like a loop, circling through the same ideas and beliefs over and over. When they stay in your head, they keep your thinking cluttered, and there is no opportunity to set them aside and look at them. Writing things down in a journal is like clearing out any spiderwebs in your head.

When you understand how your disconnected eating patterns have reaffirmed your fears, you've immediately removed the driving force to eat in a disconnected way. These stories and your fears no longer have to dictate your choices.

CLARITY PRACTICE: ACKNOWLEDGING YOUR WORTH

Disconnected eating was a practice you started and continued so you could fix your body. You and your body don't need fixing, though. Nothing is broken. You'll know this in your heart when you've connected to your true essence.

When I first started practicing yoga, I only knew namaste to be something we all said after class. We put our palms together, placed them to our forehead, and bowed. I followed along, only because it felt like a benign ritual. With more education, I understood namaste to mean, "The light in me honors and bows to the light in you. When you are in this place in you and I am in this place in me, together we are one."

This light, which we all have within us, is something I could relate to. As a mother, I can see my children in their individual beautiful brilliance. Yet I had to consider, Does every human being have this light within them? Beings with different religions, nationalities, sexual preferences and identities, abilities, and colors? Yes. Does the light exist no matter what our bodies look like? Hell, yes. Does this light exist no matter what people do and what choices they make? Yes, as we are each born with a divine essence, and that light does not require us to prove our worth, justify ourselves, or look or act a certain way.

When we connect to and acknowledge this divine light within us, the fears we've been believing just become an illusion. Like a cloud, fears inhibit our ability to see our own light. You are whole and complete and perfect. This acknowledgment is a deep knowing that we are not our mistakes, we are not our flaws. We are not even our successes.

Our divine light can't be measured, but the peace we feel in our life is a direct indication of how we acknowledge this light.

Up until this point, disconnected eating practices have removed us from the connection to our own light.

You know that for yourself. Consider how you feel about yourself in your eating patterns. Do they leave you feeling the brilliance and wholeness that I'm describing? No. Far from it. Your own experience is enough to know that.

Practice: Acknowledging Your Worth

Sit comfortably and take a few breaths in and out of your nose. Ground your body. Bring your awareness to the base of your spine. Imagine in that area the glow of a bright white light. When you have a vision of it, allow it to migrate up your spine and down your legs. With a few breaths, let this light fill your body. Notice how the light warms you and fills you with clarity. I learned this practice from Jon Gabriel and found it both comforting and empowering.

Practice this daily.

<u>Bonus Practice</u>: During this simple meditation, a mantra can help to anchor your mind. Use a few words that resonate with you. Some that may feel right are: I am light. I am love. I am truth. I am whole. I am complete.

I'm asking you to believe that this light exists within you. Consider being open to a faith where you don't need to fight against your feelings of unworthiness or work to dispute them. Instead, your faith in your own divine essence is simply acknowledging that you are divinely placed here on earth, that you are meant to be here. You don't need to achieve anything during your time here to earn this light—it's in you and never goes away. You can spend your days living however you'd like to live. It's your choice. However, why not acknowledge and connect to this light? When you do, you'll learn to rely and depend on yourself with great depth and wisdom.

Your next step is to stop working toward fixing something that's not broken by choosing to connect with your truth, time and time again. "Your truth" may seem elusive, but it's simply the loving source that sits within you.

When you choose your brilliance over your brokenness, you will start choosing to connect with yourself. Over, and over, and over again.

CHAPTER SIXTEEN

Choice

Now that you have personal insight into how your patterns around food and your body developed, it's important to recognize the choices you have in each moment. The principle of choice is practicing undoing many of the patterns that have kept that disconnected eating in place. Practicing the principle of choice is so powerful because it offers you a wider option of possible actions. The principle of choice is the power center of the Connected Eating System.

You may have seen the popular meme of twin boys of an alcoholic father. Both boys grew up in the same household under their father's rage, abuse, and alcoholism. As the boys grew up and became adults, one never drank a day in his life, while the other became an alcoholic, just like his father. Both boys justified their actions with, "My father was an alcoholic; what choice do I have?"

One son believed he was destined to follow in his father's footsteps. The other saw his father's choices as a lesson of what not to do. Each son understood the power of his own choice, or the lack thereof.

"I had no other choice" is an indicator of disconnected eating patterns. When done in a disconnected way, eating can often feel like it's happening on autopilot. If there is a plate of food in front of you, you may automatically eat the whole thing, without regard to how full you are. If it's lunchtime, you may automatically eat the salad you made for yourself that morning, even if it's a cold and rainy day and you could easily get a bowl of warm soup in the cafeteria at work. And, without much thinking, if there is a plate of cookies on the table at a networking event, you may find yourself munching on one without realizing whether you wanted it or were hungry for it.

As part of disconnected eating, we've lost sight of the choices we've been making because we've been reacting instead of acting mindfully with intention.

The principle of choice allows you to reclaim your power: power that you've either given away or forgot you even had. It's not about self-control or trying to muscle your way into making the right choice. The principle of choice runs deeper than just choosing based on how we think we should be choosing (for weight loss). **The principle of choice, when practiced within the Connected Eating System, gives you several options, each of which can be evaluated based on what aligns best with how you feel at the time, how you want to feel, and how you want to nourish your body.**

CHOICE PRACTICE:
LETTING GO OF CRITICISM

The voice of disconnected eating is critical and judgmental. We scold and berate ourselves with thoughts like, "I can't believe I ate that," "I'm so disgusting," "I'll never lose weight," "I'm so lazy and pathetic," and, "What's wrong with me?" Your thoughts have been bullying you, and now it's time to introduce a compassionate voice. At times it may be firm, at times it may be gentle. As you practice connected eating, you'll start to notice the difference between these critical and compassionate voices.

Using the principle of awareness, practice noticing your thoughts to witness how often this critical voice comes up for you—not just around your food choices but also at home, in the office, and in your relationships.

Practice: Noticing the Critical Voice

Journal out your critical voice. Take the time to get its thoughts out of your head and onto paper so they don't have to keep haunting you.

When your critical and judgmental voice comes up, you always have a choice to believe it or not. After all, thoughts are just thoughts. They aren't necessarily the truth. Just because you think something doesn't mean you need to believe it or act on it. You may even ask yourself, "What's the point in criticizing myself?"

Bonus Practice: When you notice the critic, welcome her in. You can even respond to her with, "Thanks for sharing," "That's interesting," or, "I hear you."

CHOICE PRACTICE:
USING PRESENT-TIME EATING

One of the amazing practices of connected eating is present-time eating. Present-time eating is eating when your body truly desires food, choosing a food that will make it feel the way you want to feel, while enjoying and being present for every bite.

Hungry at 10:00 a.m.? Take the time to make something that will energize you, that will taste good, and that you will fully enjoy for the moment you are in. Those decisions are made in the moment and aren't planned.

When you finish, let your meal be finished too. There's no need to think about it or consider it again. No need to rehash it or think about whether you should have eaten differently.

For dieters who have learned to plan meals in advance, bring their own food to events or parties, or eat before they go out to avoid eating the wrong thing, present-time eating is a powerful practice. It comes over time as you start to trust in yourself.

Practice: Giving Yourself the Gift of Present-Time Eating

This practice can alter so much of our energy, as we will know how to responsively sit for a meal, thoroughly enjoy it, know when to stop eating, and then move on with our day. **Connected eating means we can free ourselves up without worrying about and planning what and how much we will eat.** It feels liberating, often like you've reclaimed your life.

CHOICE PRACTICE: RECOGNIZING CRAVINGS

There is no doubting how persistent and determined cravings can be. They sit in the front of our minds, demanding our attention. In connected eating, cravings aren't something to avoid or be fearful of. Instead, they are just another signal or cue, something to tune us back into our bodies.

Years before I practiced connected eating, I remember craving a Hershey's Kiss one day, and I made a choice to eat the little chocolate. When I went back to the kitchen to grab a handful of them, and when I unwrapped each one and put it in my mouth, each of those actions was a choice I'd made. At the time, I hadn't acknowledged the choice I was making. I walked back and forth to the kitchen from the living room like I was sleepwalking, eating without realizing what I was doing. In my healing process, I had to realize that every time I ate something, I was making a choice. Every time I contemplated eating something and didn't, I had to have the awareness that I was making a choice.

If you eat in a disconnected manner, eating too much or eating a forbidden food has been viewed as the bad or wrong choice. Now, your view of what's good or bad can be changed. With connected eating, there is no bad or wrong choice. It's simply a choice you are actively making.

With this in mind, why would we want to ignore our cravings? Why would we want to wish them away?

When we are in connection with our body and in partnership with the sensations that often emerge, cravings don't become something to avoid. Instead, they become something to welcome and to witness.

Recognizing the craving is recognizing that we are craving something, often something that food cannot fill. When we choose to fill an emotional void when we are not hungry, there is no amount of food that will fill us up. As you start to shift your relationship with food, let your cravings be a glorious sign that you need something, something that you may have never given yourself before.

Practice: Being with Cravings

Drop into your body and ask, What is this craving telling me? Assuming it has words, what does it want to share?

Give yourself permission to eat if you choose to eat. Like the noticing your feelings clarity practice, set a timer for five minutes and give yourself the time to be with the craving first. Afterward, you can revisit your choice. At any given point in time, eating is an option. I find that when it's an available option for us, it's easier to make other choices.

Don't push or shove your cravings away. Like a beacon of light allowing you to easily see the path in front of you, let your cravings be your guidance on how to nourish yourself.

By trying to fix the craving, we are trying to fix something that's not broken. The craving isn't the problem, because we aren't the problem. The craving is just a signal that something needs attention. When we call something a problem, we want to fix it. This craving is simply your body's way of drawing attention to something.

Bonus Practice: Food has been such a source of comfort for us, so why would we want to give that up? What would happen to us if we didn't have food? It would be like riding a bike without training wheels if we had never ridden a bike before. This is why we approach this process with great compassion and great tenacity.

CHOICE PRACTICE: CARING FOR YOURSELF

The practice of connected eating isn't just about food; it's also about how we care for ourselves with and without food. When we've cared for ourselves, giving ourselves what we need and treating ourselves kindly, how we eat doesn't need to fill any missing gaps. If we've been eating to fill a void when we've been engaging in disconnected eating, we know that no amount of food will make us truly feel better.

Caring for yourself is affirming the care you want for yourself. It's time to create daily practices to affirm how much your body and your self is worth caring for. Building your solid foundation isn't just nice to have, it's a requirement. You don't have to earn it; instead, doing things that connect you back to yourself is what every person does to be the best they can be in their body.

Caring for yourself is important so you can have the energy for new habits. There are many contributors to our energy levels. Sleep is an obvious one. But it's not the only one. I know I always feel better when I'm well hydrated, when I've spent time outside, and when I've given myself some downtime. I call this practice creating a solid daily foundation. It's time to stop running yourself ragged. By keeping yourself busy, you don't have time for yourself, and you neglect your own sleep and time for play.

Practice: Creating a Daily Care Practice

Make a list of all the actions you can take that will make you feel better. It's not about burning calories or doing the "should" things. It's about finding things that nourish you. Quilting, painting, grabbing that mindless and easy read with your favorite soft blanket, practicing a musical instrument—these are the things that create a solid foundation, ones that make you feel great.

From the outside, creating a solid daily foundation may seem simple. Practice choosing at least three things every day that improve how you feel in your body.

Bonus Practice: When we make this a habit, noticing how we feel and what we do to improve our well-being is an important connection to make. We will know what we need to do every day to have a steady flow of energy. Become aware of how caring for yourself shifts how your awareness of your thoughts, feelings, and body sensations. Notice how your connection to your body changes with the amount of time you take to care for yourself. You can even journal about it.

When you've taken the time to care for yourself, your inner source starts to emerge. Like it's been awakened, acknowledged, and respected, a new energy source will start offering you its guidance. This is when it's time to start listening.

CHAPTER SEVENTEEN

Listening

Where principle of choice is like erasing a chalkboard so it's clean and green, the principle of listening provides us space to write something brand new. Listening is the principle of acknowledging a new mechanism, one that comes from your own intuition, to guide you. The principle of listening is about recognizing your new power source and using it as a guide.

Have you ever made a decision, one you debated over and over, and knew immediately it was the wrong one? You may have even shared with a close friend, "I knew in my gut I should have chosen otherwise." Listening is about recognizing your "gut" when she speaks to you. When we've ignored this power source, we've prioritized outside messages, expectations we think others have for us, and old and often painful thought patterns.

Listening is about hearing your own internal wisdom and following through on her guidance.

Connected eating choices are informed by our body, our emotions, and our intuition. With the listening principle, there will be an emergence. You will be coming forward, as the whole you. This guidance is something you've always had. You've been walking around with it, and now you'll begin to recognize it. You'll begin to call upon it. You'll begin to require that this guidance is strongly considered when you choose what to eat, when to eat, and how to eat. The more you work with the listening principle, the stronger your power source will become.

LISTENING PRACTICE: EMBRACING YOUR BODY

Your body is an extension of yourself, not the core of yourself. The old saying, "Don't judge a book by its cover" rings true here. We are so much more than our cover, no matter if our cover is a size 4, size 14, or size 24.

For years, I would pass by a mirror or a reflection in a window and size my body up. Was it too big? Did my thighs look too fat in what I was wearing? I'd be measuring myself up based on what was reflected back at me.

Changing how you think about your body may take time, or it may take an instant when you recognize the truth. Your body is something to honor and cherish. You've gotten it all wrong. Now it's time to apologize to it and ask it what it needs and what it wants to share with you.

As I began to go through my own healing process, I had to go toward those parts of my body that I had been criticizing, wanting to hide, and wishing to change.

I'd put my hands on my thighs and belly and feel thickness, curves, and extra. When the judgment came up, I wanted to pull away. I kept practicing feeling my thighs objectively and letting them be exactly as they were. It was as if my memory and judgments around what an acceptable body was had been erased, and I could just feel parts of myself that I had been gifted. Flashes of memories came up. The marathon I ran, the hikes I finished, climbing stairs with one of my babies on my hip.

When I could simply notice my thighs for what they were and what they had offered me, I could embrace my strength and power.

Practice: Recognizing Your Body's Brilliance

Imagine you are seeing and feeling your body for the first time. No one told you your body needed to be different from what it is. In fact, you just told yourself your body is perfect, just as it is. It's perfect simply because it's yours and it's not anything different.

Look in the mirror and notice parts of your body you have taken the time to witness. Put your hands on your arms, hands, legs, thighs, breasts. Feel what's underneath your hands. Get to know your body now that you are choosing not to judge it.

Bonus Practice: What has your body offered you that you haven't acknowledged? What gifts has it given to you? Talk to your body when you catch a glimpse of her in a reflection. Take the time to journal about your experience.

It's your choice whether you love your body or not. Yours and yours only. Your body is the source of feedback, sharing with you how you feel. It's a perfect container, one that you can use to express yourself and adorn.

LISTENING PRACTICE: REPLACING BODY COMPARISON WITH COMPASSION

A few summers ago, I challenged myself. I went to the beach and paid attention to my initial reaction to every woman I saw. I noticed how easy it was for me to judge other women's bodies, comparing my own to theirs. This time, instead of just looking at the neck down, I paid attention to her face, looking at her eyes and smile. I started to notice each woman's beauty, not from what size bikini or bathing suit she was wearing, but instead by seeing all of her. How could I even judge these women? I didn't even know them, I never spoke with them. I noticed how peaceful I started to feel in my own body on the beach.

Our judgment of other women's bodies is really judgment of our own. The critical thoughts running through our minds aren't just criticizing our bodies; they're criticizing other bodies as well. By changing our minds about other bodies we see, we can change our minds about our own.

Practice: Witnessing the Beauty in All Women
Do the exercise I did at the beach for yourself. Anyplace is fine—while shopping, at work, at a sporting event, or at the beach. Is this something you feel excited about doing, or do you feel resistance toward it?

Bonus Practice: Take the time to journal about your experience and ask yourself these questions:

- What if you didn't have to compare yourself to a former version of yourself?

- What if you didn't have to compare yourself to others?

- How has your body protected you and kept you safe?

LISTENING PRACTICE: CULTIVATING YOUR VITALITY

Dropping your attention away from your thinking brain to your body takes some practice. As you start to appreciate your body for how valuable it is and how wise it is, going to it more and more will become second nature.

Your body holds the source of your vitality. Starting to notice the right amount of food and what kinds of food cultivates this vitality is a powerful practice. Remember the hunger and fullness continuum from our awareness practice? You've noticed where you are when you typically start and stop eating, so now it's time to bring more mindfulness around how your body feels when you eat when you are hungry enough and how you stop eating when you are content.

Practice: Finding Out the Ideal What, How Much, and When of Eating

After you've grounded yourself in your body, notice your hunger. At what point on the continuum does food taste the best? At what point do you feel most excited to eat? At what point do you feel you can eat most calmly?

For me, I'm generally between 3 and 4. If I go past 3, I tend to eat too quickly.

Notice at what point you feel best stopping eating. You may feel most satisfied at a 5, or it may be more like a 5 1/2.

Knowing your own vitality is knowing how your body feels best when you nourish it with food.

Beginning with the end in mind is a powerful practice. How do you want to feel after you've finished eating? Being clear with ourselves around how we want to feel in our body is so important because it's a reflection of what we want.

Bonus Practice: Having conversations with your body is a beautiful practice of asking questions and patiently listening for a response. Your body has offered you information over the years, but you've either negotiated with it in your mind or intentionally dismissed it, or perhaps you have been too busy to listen. That's okay. The good news is that this skill of awareness will come back to you quickly.

Start your day, every day, by intentionally having a conversation with your body. After a few deep rounds of grounding breaths, take a few moments to scan for energy and sensation. Ask your whole body:

What would make me feel better today?

What can I do to increase my energy? Where is my vitality? How does it feel in my body?

Your body holds more than information on how hungry and full you really are. It also holds sensations around how you are feeling. It also holds your intuition, an ability to guide you instinctively. This is where you come to life fully.

LISTENING PRACTICE: OFFERING YOURSELF FORGIVENESS

We've beaten ourselves up for going off plan, failing at our dieting, and eating emotionally. Even though we've believed getting mad at ourselves or even being disgusted with ourselves motivates us to change our behavior, it's never worked to change how we eat.

Up until this point, you probably couldn't imagine forgiving yourself for every time you overate, underate, and ate so much your belly was screaming at you. Forgiving ourselves for eating half a box of Girl Scout cookies could mean we may eat a whole box next time. We may lose our discipline and focus. After all, if we forgive ourselves, we've let ourselves off the hook.

I watched how I felt and what I did when I beat myself up after a binge. I felt worse. I was more rigid with myself. It was impossible for me to do anything right. With every binge, the fear of more weight gain was met with a need to eat fewer calories and exercise more. I had this idea of a perfect day, and I couldn't do it. I always failed. Each mistake led me to higher standards for myself, standards that felt impossible for me to reach.

Forgiveness gives you permission to continue to do what you want to do. Instant forgiveness offers you an opportunity to fully own your actions, to accept them, and to take responsibility for them. When we beat ourselves up, the martyr in us comes out. We must be punished, and we make sure that we punish ourselves by removing certain foods and maintaining the lowest of calories. We punish ourselves with the strictest of standards and brutal self-talk.

Without forgiveness, you will continue to reinforce perfectionism and the destructive all-or-nothing mentality that keeps disconnected eating in place. Forgiveness makes room for us. It's required to stop the binge cycle.

Practice: Giving the Gift of Forgiveness

Journal the answers to these questions: What needs forgiving? If your body was your best friend, what would you need to share with her? What does she need to hear from you?

Bonus Practice: The moment you know the so-called mistake is made, smile. Maybe even laugh. Instead of engaging in the heaviness of a mistake, welcome the lightness of seeing that you can take full ownership of your choice and also choose intently next time.

Bonus Practice: The ho'oponopono Hawaiian prayer is simple and beautiful:

I'm sorry. Please forgive me. Thank you. I love you.

As you say this quietly to yourself, bring yourself into your mind's eye.

Over time, consider this same prayer for someone you may want to forgive. Forgiveness is a practice that allows you to release the judgment you may be making against others as well as yourself.

———

When you practice the principle of listening, you start to uncover the truth and connect with your own brilliance. Now, you know this brilliance is worth illuminating. Next, you will practice the principle of alignment. The first step in alignment is giving yourself permission to free your mind from food, to trust your body, and to love yourself.

CHAPTER EIGHTEEN

Alignment

It's one thing to know what to do; it's another to actually do it. The principle of alignment is hearing your new voice and guidance and following through by being in action. The principle of alignment is the most impactful of all the practices, and it's the one that sets a new direction for every other area of your life, not just how you eat and how you relate to your body.

The Dictionary.com definition of alignment is "a state of agreement or cooperation among persons, groups, nations, etc. with a common cause or viewpoint." Alignment exists when two people work together with similar values, purpose, and intention. In disconnected eating, we've been aligning with a part of us that's not serving our best interests. The part that is fearful and believes we aren't enough. The part that believes we have to fix our body. And the part of us that has had thoughts of food take over our lives.

Creating alignment is the process of getting to know yourself and creating habits and actions that are consistent with your truest self.

For years, I ran multiple businesses: an accounting consulting firm, a yoga studio, and my transformational coaching business. Even as I write these words, I recognize the insanity of trying to handle all this responsibility. Eventually I let go of the accounting firm and yoga studio, or, you could say, they let go of me. Yet it took me years to see what I had outgrown and to claim what energized me and lit me up. My body offered me this insight. I was often exhausted and frustrated when I worked in spreadsheets and generated reports for clients. I felt grounded when I worked with coaching clients, and I also felt shifts taking place between us that weren't of my doing, but of something bigger.

Moving into just one business meant I needed to do two things. I had to give myself permission to work in a business I loved, even if it felt risky and uncertain. I also had to trust myself and know that I could create my business and be successful in it.

I notice when I've made aligned choices, I feel like I'm on solid ground. I know that I've connected more to myself rather than betrayed myself. And thanks to that, I move through those choices easily, without any further reflection or contemplation. I don't dwell on what I just ate for the rest of the day. I don't need to. I don't plan any future meals. I don't need to. I trust myself to make the choice in the moment. That's what alignment can bring you.

Alignment creates a synergy, one that can make you feel like your life is both safe to navigate and also unpredictable. When we're aligned, the concept of being in control takes on a new meaning. We aren't dictating the outcome of events with our own agenda, but instead, we have the faith and confidence that no matter what gets tossed our way, we can stay connected to ourselves. A relaxed resilience develops, so every part of us wins. The part of you that wants to feel safe and in control wins. And the part of you that wants to feel free and enjoy life wins. Alignment is the beautiful win-win.

As you work with alignment, you'll find that it's really an exploration of what suits you best in any given moment. We are always making choices and reacting to our own ideals, assumptions, and values. The question is, Are those ours or someone else's? What are you aligning yourself to? And when it comes to how we treat our bodies, what does it take to give ourselves full permission to eat what we want to eat? How do we know which foods nourish us and fill us, and which ones deplete us?

ALIGNMENT PRACTICE:
GIVING YOURSELF PERMISSION

Sipping on iced tea in an outdoor cafe, I noticed three older women, a few tables over, enjoying ice cream sundaes. It was early afternoon on a warmer than usual September day.

They laughed together in what looked like a steady and easy conversation. I could sense their comfort and ease. To say they were quietly confident would be an understatement.

What came first for these three women: the permission to eat the sundae, or the permission to receive pleasure? What comes first for us, the ability to trust ourselves around any food, or the ability to trust ourselves to nourish ourselves and our body in a perfect way? Could they be receiving more nourishment from their companionship, connection, and conversation than from the sundaes?

As you work with the practice of alignment, you will be establishing your own way of eating, moving, and ultimately nourishing yourself. You will have trusted yourself enough to know that you really are the only one who can hold the answers to: What should I eat? How should I move? When should I sleep? What do I need? These can only be asked of yourself. You are the only one who could possibly know the answers.

Practice: Redefining Food as Nourishment

What food have you been withholding from eating? A piece of delicious chocolate cake from that amazing bakery around the corner? The freshest strawberries from the farmers market?

Have you been depriving yourself of rest? What would it be like if you slept an extra hour tomorrow?

Giving yourself permission is seeing how you've been holding yourself back from simple pleasures and necessary nourishment.

When we were engaged in disconnected eating, food held tremendous meaning. It was an avenue for us to either gain weight or lose weight. Now, your practice is letting food be lovely. **Enjoying the food you love is possible when you do it with all your attention, with no guilt or shame, and from a place of complete connection to the signals of your body.** It's all about giving yourself permission.

Let's redefine food from merely being calories, something that's good or bad, something to avoid or eat more of, something processed or whole. Instead, let food be what it is. A source that can energize you and do wonders to make your body come alive, and something you can thoroughly and completely enjoy.

Bonus Practice: Get out your journal and pen. Take some time with what you've been withholding from yourself.

- What would you be doing if you weren't afraid of being fully seen?

- What would you be doing if you weren't afraid of failing?

- Is there anything in the way of giving yourself permission to be happy, just as you are?

ALIGNMENT PRACTICE: CULTIVATING GRATITUDE

You've heard about the power of gratitude practice, and now you are hearing about it again. Noticing what you appreciate in your life is a way of identifying what you value. Gratitude is the practice of directing your energy toward what you appreciate in life and want more of. When you are grateful for something, you notice the positive, the strength, and the beauty. The more you place your energy around what you love, the more your love will grow.

Practice: Experiencing the Magic of Gratitude

For this practice, simply write down at least three things you're grateful for every day. Always include something about your body and food. Consider these questions to start you off:

- Do you appreciate that your feet can take you from one place to the other?

- Are you grateful for the meal you prepared last night and how it left you feeling so content?

- Are you grateful for the fresh eggs you enjoyed for breakfast from the farmers market?

A gratitude practice is one that will benefit all areas of your life and only requires that you acknowledge what you appreciate.

Bonus Practice: Say it out loud. Share your gratitude with your family, friends, and coworkers. Start to witness the magic of what happens when you share what you are grateful for. Gratitude is contagious—the more you share it, the more it spreads.

Notice if parts of your life start to change, like extra praise from someone at work, a beautiful chat with a loved one, or an unexpected gift of money.

ALIGNMENT PRACTICE:
RECOGNIZING PLEASURE, JOY, AND FUN

When engaged in connected eating, we've found the little girl in us who was allowed to play, laugh, enjoy life, and have fun. Disconnected eating can feel like a part-time job. It's heavy, it's hard, and we can feel the weight of the world on our shoulders.

We can enjoy pleasure in our life, and we can also enjoy pleasure in food. Eating is enjoyable! Now that food is not the enemy, taking the time to thoroughly enjoy it makes our lives richer and sweeter.

I had a fantastic meal with my two best girlfriends on a cold winter evening. We were in a gorgeous hotel, overlooking the water, in the best seats available—right in front of the fireplace in these super-comfy, red velvet chairs. It was perfect. I couldn't help notice how we were eating, taking bites of our food calmly and enjoying the flavors.

That evening, I began a beautiful connected eating practice before I took one bite of food. It started when I considered the menu and chose what I wanted to eat based on how the food would nourish and fulfill me. Before it came, I grounded myself in my body, taking a few breaths that allowed me to feel my wholeness. Then, I took each bite, noticing my experience of eating. This connected eating practice allowed me to experience not just the nourishment of the food but also the nourishment of my friendships, of our easy conversations, and of the warmth of the fire.

Food can taste delicious. Real, fresh, sour, sweet. It can warm our body and make it come alive. It can be so pleasurable, if we let it. And when we eat for taste, for enjoyment—when our senses take in every sniff, bite, lick, and ounce of it—we won't be needing more. By fully engaging in the enjoyment of eating, a few bites may leave you completely satisfied.

Practice: Playing

Letting yourself have fun and enjoy the pleasures of life is a necessity. We've been tossing our fun and joy aside, believing that maybe we aren't allowed to have it, or we can't have too much, or we'll feel guilty if we do.

But now, we can align with this part of us that we have been neglecting. **I notice the more I receive joy and pleasure with play, with restoration, and in other areas of my life, food doesn't have to play that part.** I don't need food to be anything other than nourishment.

Ask yourself:

- How can I play more in my life?

- When and where can I intentionally have more fun?

- What are ways I can enjoy food more?

- What foods have I been depriving myself of for sheer pleasure?

You've given yourself permission; now you're going to be more proactive and incorporate pleasure and fun consistently in your life.

Bonus Practice: Take out your journal and pen. What has held you back from joy, pleasure, and fun in the past? Do you have a story that you've created around needing to earn your fun? Or are these ideas new to you, something that was never modeled to you as a child and therefore never considered?

ALIGNMENT PRACTICE: CREATING A VISION AND PURPOSE

We've been peeling away all the beliefs and habits that have created our disconnected eating. It's almost like we've been taking off layers like an onion, getting to our center. All the layers have been holding us back. Now the question is: What propels us forward?

You have a choice in your future. Disconnected eating sucks the life out of future possibilities. Creating a vision for yourself can be so fun and exciting. Allowing yourself to visualize the unknown and seemingly impossible is a powerful affirmation in acknowledging your own worth.

Disconnected eating has distracted us from something bigger that lives within us. When we recognize this bigger calling, this greater purpose, the process and act of stepping toward that purpose will call upon us to be more of who we need to be to serve out our purpose.

Your purpose is something that moves you personally. Your purpose is unique to you, as it may not move your best friend, your sister, or your college roommate. But it moves you to your core. You can identify your purpose by noticing what brings you to life. Your heart beats faster, all your senses turn on, and you feel light.

Stepping into our purpose requires something of us, and if we have habits, beliefs, and thoughts that aren't in alignment with this, they will need to drop away. If they don't, we will be stopped, confronted, and resistant. Our ability to go far toward our purpose depends 100 percent on alignment—body, mind, and spirit.

Practice: Connecting with Your Passions and Purpose

Get out your journal and pen, then answer these questions:

- What breaks your heart?

- If you could change one thing in the world, what would it be?

- What are your talents, life experiences, and passions that no one else can offer?

Be interested in finding out these answers. If the answers don't come right away, keep asking yourself these questions. Connecting with your spark may take some patience and diligence.

Bonus Practice: Take the time to design your vision for how you want to nourish yourself and the habits you want to create. Consider how you want to take the time to cook yourself nutritious meals. How else in your life can you feel joy and pleasure? By doing work that you love, you say? By swimming in the warm ocean, you say? By climbing into warm, soft sheets at the end of the day, you say? Yes, please, you say?

Design a statement that summarizes what you want, then create a visual of your future self.

Play out this visual of a typical day in this newly designed life in your mind. As you do, feel how you want to feel, as if this isn't just a visualization, but reality.

Bonus Practice: Consider your own practices, how you connect with yourself daily, so you can show up as your best, clearest, brightest, most energetic and connected self. Feeling good in your body and making choices that serve your body best are in alignment with your purpose.

- What are the habits that support you fulfilling your purpose?

- What habits will dull you and stop you from fulfilling your purpose?

Find your purpose, and then your goals will easily fall into place to fulfill that purpose.

There you have it. The five principles in the Connected Eating System are designed to do one simple thing: bring you back to yourself. I've shared some of my favorite practices with you, ones that my clients and I have found to be most impactful. Consider each practice and bonus practice as a step. A step you deliberately take to guide you in the right direction. I invite you to practice each of them a few times to find out which ones work best for you.

As you practice connected eating, you will get to know yourself, your passions, and your purpose, and you will also recognize your brilliance. Following your purpose with alignment is an affirming process. As we change how we eat, the food we choose, and how we look at our body, it's like finding a perfect pair of jeans. Do we like dark wash or light? High-waisted or low? Straight leg, cropped, or bootcut?

When we can feel what feels right, our sense of our own self and what's important to us becomes clearer. This is why alignment doesn't impact just our relationship with food—it also reframes our whole relationship with ourselves.

CHAPTER NINETEEN

What's Next

My sincerest desire is that you now understand two things. First, you know the real reasons why food has been a struggle for you. And, second, you know that practicing connected eating and ultimately honoring, listening to, and trusting your body is the only way for you to be truly free around food.

YOUR BODY IS YOUR HOME

As young children, we knew our body instinctively. It told us when we needed rest, it told us when we were upset and angry, and it told us when our belly had just enough food. Our body was a neutral yet obvious part of us. Our body was simply a vehicle in which we knew how to express ourselves.

While writing this book, I had lunch with Nancy. Remember that I was on the cross-country team in college? Nancy was on our track team. We were chatting about what sports our kids were playing. One of her kids, begrudgingly to Nancy, had no interest in running. She shared with me a conversation she had with her nine-year-old daughter. "I told her, 'Well, it's a good thing you're thin.'" She smiled as she shared this with me, while I sat stunned and speechless.

Over lunch at a local cafe, the message of required thinness was spreading. It spreads from mother to daughter, friend to friend, TV actor to TV viewer, Instagram account to Instagram account. *Undetected.* The message is embedded in Nancy's mind, my mind, and yours. It's in the fabric of our culture.

This message has been the origin of the disconnection you have from your body. When we couldn't help but believe the message that we needed to be thin, our view of our body changed. Our body needs to look a certain way for us to feel good about ourselves. By holding our body as a way to value ourselves, we disconnect from it.

Now you know. Start by clearly and confidently identifying and dismissing these messages, past and future. By doing so, you will be affirming the truth about yourself. Your body doesn't need to be a way to get the approval of others, fit in, and be accepted. Your body is something to appreciate. A gift while you walk along this earth. A home for your energy and your soul. You knew that on the day you were born, and it's time to remind yourself of this truth.

FOOD NOURISHES

Our culture is as obsessed with thinness as it is with food. We've been told to diet, restrict certain foods, and forbid others because they are dirty and disgusting. We've been told to eat "clean." Yet we hear messages that food can comfort us as a source of fun and celebration. The contradiction is freakin' insane, and this is what I know: You and I have given our power away to food. We've been at its mercy, and it's robbed us of time, energy, and headspace. This needs to end, right now. We don't need another recipe or another cookbook. We don't need another supposed expert to tell us what to eat.

It's time to stop seeking a solution outside of us. It's time to listen to what's going on *inside.*

Standing in your power around food is like standing in your own power around religion and politics. It's personal. And it's no one's business but your own. You now know the truth about your body. It's time for you and your body to choose to eat. You've only been struggling with food because you've been rebelling against someone else's rules, you've been serving another master that is not your own, and you've been fighting yourself daily. This has created a clear disconnection.

It's time to face and listen to our expertise—and, in turn, take full responsibility for ourselves and our bodies. This is the beautiful opportunity you've been waiting for. When you follow your own wisdom, you're in alignment with yourself around how you want to feel. You don't need discipline or motivation to eat in a way that nourishes you. Instead, fueling yourself is simply a way of life.

READY TO FEEL

We are emotional creatures. We make decisions and act based on how we feel. For years, I engaged in disconnected eating because I simply wanted to avoid how I felt. I thought I was feeling sad and ate a bowl of ice cream. But really, I was starting to anticipate the beginning of feeling sad and wanted to distract myself with a bowl of ice cream.

Does this make me disordered? Compulsive? An overeater? Addicted?

Believing we are any of these labels and staying in the cycle of distracting ourselves from necessary feelings continues disconnected eating.

It's okay that we've comforted ourselves with food. It's okay that we are afraid of how we feel. It's okay to feel. We aren't broken, and we don't need to be fixed for simply being human.

My healing road required me to be really compassionate with myself. I had to stop blaming myself or feeling bad that I was so angry. I needed to soften around my sadness and know that it wasn't going to pull me into a state of everlasting depression. I'm committed to walking this road. My feelings don't need to be justified or defended. I just let them come. I keep letting go of the belief that something is wrong with me, and I do my best to welcome how I feel. I know now that it's just as easy to believe we are broken as it is to believe we aren't.

By practicing connected eating, you will practice being with yourself as you feel what you feel. This is one of the most remarkable things you can do for yourself. Food will no longer be a distraction. Your body will be an ally. And you will honor yourself deeply by being with every sensation, every tear, every sob and scream. It's glorious. You'll see.

ONE MORE THING

I'll toss in one last thing I want you to know. Actually, the most important one.

You now know why you've really struggled with food. You now know how you can make your way back to freeing yourself around food by connecting with your truest self. Your body and your natural wisdom are both yours to connect with. They are only one breath away.

You have everything you need, right now, to move toward this freedom.

You've been hungry for this deep connection with yourself. Practicing awareness, clarity, choice, listening, and alignment will wake you up, connect you deeply, and set you on a path to design your life in a way that fits you best. You have this insight and power residing deep within you. Self-trust will emerge from the practice of connected eating, and when that happens, your struggles with food and your body will fall away. Your mind will be free, and you will trust your body and value yourself completely, just the way you are. This is the journey to satisfying your hunger, my friend. Making your way back to yourself is a beautiful process. I'm with you every step of the way. Ready? Let's begin.

♥

Endnotes

1. "General Statistics," National Eating Disorders Association, accessed February 13, 2019, https://www.nationaleatingdisorders.org/general-statistics.

2. Chris Iliades, "Stats and Facts about Depression in America," Everyday Health, last modified January 23, 2013, https://www.everydayhealth.com/hs/major-depression/depression-statistics/.

3. "The Incredible Shrinking Miss America," CBS News, January 31, 2002, https://www.cbsnews.com/

4. Michael Dawson, "The Marketing Race: Straight from the Horse's Mouth," The Consumer Trap, May 8, 2008, https://www.consumertrap.com/tag/yankelovich/.

5. Pamela Peeke, "Just What IS an Average Woman's Size Anymore?," WebMD Blog, January 25, 2010, https://blogs.webmd.com/from-our-archives/20100125/just-what-is-an-average-womans-size-anymore.

6. Pinterest, posted by Chris Gillespie in Vintage Ads and Products board on or around May 2019, https://www.pinterest.com/pin/320670435943556834/

7. "About Let's Move," LetsMove.gov (archived), https://lets-move.obamawhitehouse.archives.gov/about.

8. Mark Memmott, "Lululemon Founder: Our Pants Won't Work for Some Women," The Two-Way, NPR.org, November 7, 2013, https://www.npr.org/sections/thetwo-way/2013/11/07/243706174/lululemon-founder-our-pants-wont-work-for-some-women.

9. Kelsey Miller, "Study: Most Girls Start Dieting by Age 8," Refinery29, January 26, 2015, https://www.refinery29.com/en-us/2015/01/81288/children-dieting-body-image.

10. Stuart Wolpert, "Dieting Does Not Work, UCLA researchers report," press release, UCLA, April 3, 2007, http://newsroom.ucla.edu/releases/Dieting-Does-Not-Work-UCLA-Researchers-7832.

11. Kathryn Doyle, "6 Years after The Biggest Loser, Metabolism Is Slower and Weight Is Back Up," Scientific American, May 11, 2016, https://www.scientificamerican.com/article/6-years-after-the-biggest-loser-metabolism-is-slower-and-weight-is-back-up/.

12. Jamie Ducharme, "About Half of Americans Say They're Trying to Lose Weight," Time, July 12, 2018, http://time.com/5334532/weight-loss-americans/

13. David Garner, "Body Image in America: Survey Results," Psychology Today, last updated September 14, 2017, https://www.psychologytoday.com/us/articles/199702/body-image-in-america-survey-results.

Before You Go

A QUICK FAVOR

Would you please leave a review
of this book on Amazon?

It's important that this essential message gets
shared with as many women who are struggling
with food and their body image as possible.

Your review will help this book reach more readers.

Thank you for sharing your opinion!
I so appreciate it.

—Tara

Acknowledgments

This book wouldn't be possible without my amazing family. They know this book as well as anyone, helped me craft the title, and patiently listened while I've ranted, raved, and even cried. I can feel them even when I don't say a word and when I've been a hundred miles away to write. I love you #whitneyfun.

Mark, you promised that you would be honest with me before we even got married, and you held that promise in my writing of this book. I love that I can rely on your honesty and that you stay calm when I'm not. I'm so incredibly grateful for your gift of love, laughter, and security. Thank you for supporting not just me as your wife, but also my passion and vision. I'm so blessed.

Ryan, thank you for getting me. I know that may be a lot for a son to offer his mother, but you do (get me), and I feel it every day. When you picked out this book cover, I was reminded that you knew the face of this book before I did. You do more than pay attention; you inspire me.

Garrett, your brilliant sixteen-year-old insight amazes me. You've challenged me in ways I could hear without feeling any criticism or judgment. Every time I asked, "Can I bounce something off you?" you were an angel, listening and reflecting along with me. Thank you. I know you don't want to be called an angel, but you really are.

Anna, you, my dearest, continue to be a bottle of hope and healing all in one beautiful mixture. I'm inspired as I see you nourish your body in the most connected way. I know, even if you don't hear me when I've asked you to clean your room, that you hear everything I say around this book and how it came to be. Thank you for seeing and hearing me. You are a love.

I know and appreciate the unquestionable strength and support of my mother and brother. If I were in a fighting match, I know they'd both be in my corner. Thank you. I love you so much.

Thank you to two women, Ann Sheybani and Carmell Clark, who saw something in me as a writer and as a transformational coach. You knew me and this book before I did, and without your clear encouragement this book may not have been possible (or may have taken many more years to finish).

Thank you to my countless friends and clients, each of whom cheered me on by simply asking, "How's your book coming along? I can't wait to read it!" Thank you for your love and accountability.

Thank you to some brilliant, creative, and meticulous editors and designers; without their contributions, this book would not be what it is today. Jennifer Hartmann, I'm so appreciative of your clear and gentle guidance and patience with me. Christina Roth, you made my message and writing even stronger. Thanks for having my back. Domini Dragoone, thanks for taking the time to get to know me and the content in this book and to capture it all so beautifully in one cover design. I had the best possible team to work with. I'm so grateful.

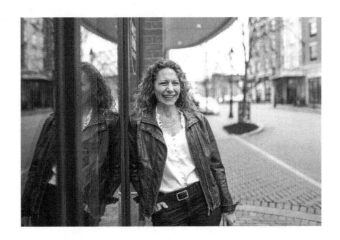

About the Author

Tara Whitney is leading a revolution of women who are creating a relationship with food and their bodies that brings them to trust themselves. Her latest book, *Hungry: Trust Your Body and Free Your Mind around Food*, offers a fresh perspective on why women have struggled with food and a path to set themselves free.

Tara is a transformational coach, author, and speaker. As a CPA, she spent over 25 years serving emerging and growing businesses with their accounting and financial needs. She has founded and grown several businesses, including an accounting consulting firm and a yoga studio. She's a Certified Intuitive Eating Counselor, Yoga Life Coach, Registered Yoga Teacher, and Level 2 Reiki Practitioner. Tara, her husband, Mark, and their three children create plenty of adventure on the Seacoast of New Hampshire and beyond. Find more about Tara at www.tara-whitney.com.